Joint Library of Ophthalmology, Moorfields Eye Hospital & UCL Institute of Ophthalmology

Library website: www.ucl.ac.uk/library/iophth
Tel: 020 7608 6814 / 020 7566 2084

To be returned on or before the date marked below

To renew your loans online, you need to go to the library catalogue http://library.ucl.ac.uk and log into My Account with your barcode number starting 028 and your 4 digit PIN

Essentials in Ophthalmology

Series Editor
Arun D. Singh

For further volumes:
http://www.springer.com/series/5332

Aniz Girach • Marc D. de Smet

Editors

Arun D. Singh

Series Editor

Diseases of the Vitreo-Macular Interface

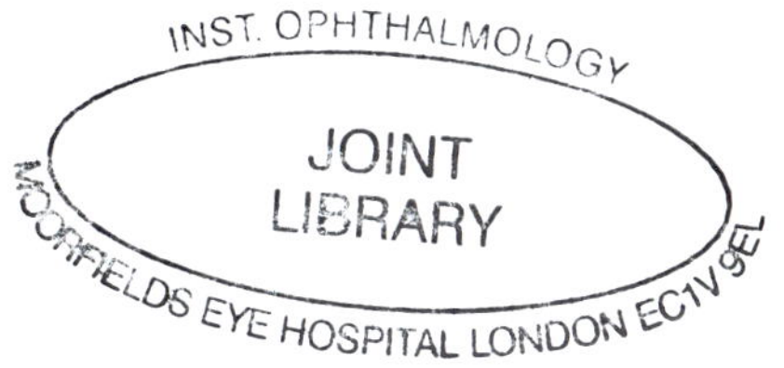

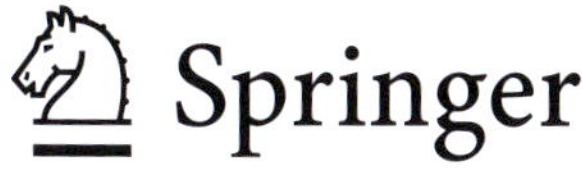

Editors
Aniz Girach, MD
ThromboGenics NV
Leuven
Belgium

Marc D. de Smet, MDCM, PhD, FRCSC
Retina and Ocular Inflammation, MIOS
Lausanne
Switzerland

Vitreoretinal Surgery Unit
Clinique de Montchoisi
Lausanne
Switzerland

Series Editor
Arun D. Singh
Depertment of Ophthalmic Oncology
Cole Eye Institute
Cleveland Clinic Foundation
Cleveland, OH
USA

ISSN 1612-3212
ISBN 978-3-642-40033-9   ISBN 978-3-642-40034-6   (eBook)
DOI 10.1007/978-3-642-40034-6
Springer Heidelberg New York Dordrecht London

Library of Congress Control Number: 2013954984

Printed on acid-free paper

Springer is part of Springer Science+Business Media (www.springer.com)

Foreword

Normal posterior vitreous detachment (PVD) occurs in everyone as we mature, but occasionally this natural process runs array and an anomalous PVD is produced leading to vitreo-macular interface (VMI) disorders. Without optical coherence tomography (OCT), our understanding of this phenomenon was limited. The advent of OCT and in small part ultrasonography has given us better insight into VMI disorders. This excellent text explores this phenomenon and its consequences in great detail. Moreover, in the past, we had only two options to treat the problem—observation and surgery. The recent approval of a vitreolysis agent has added another arrow to our quiver to attack VMI disease and its consequences. In the future, other agents or a cocktail of agents may further improve our ability to treat these common conditions.

Drs. Girach and de Smet have compiled an exceptional list of contributors who are experts in the field and who have been researching various facets of VMI diseases for years. This book begins with an overview of the disease and how it affects patients. Next, vitreous biochemistry and the pathophysiology of the vitreo-macular interface are explored. Importantly, best practices on imaging the various VMI disorders are explored in detail. Finally, methods to treat VMI disorders are discussed. Both current and future options are addressed. After reading this text, readers will have a complete understanding of VMI disorders. We are indebted to the editors and authors for delivering this much-needed reference on VMI, the first text of its kind dealing with a common potentially sight-threatening disorder.

Cleveland, USA   Peter K. Kaiser, MD

Preface

The eye is a wondrous organ. It is derived from all primeval layers of the developing embryo, each of its parts having developed specific functions constrained by the requirements of a developing eye, the provision of vision, and structural integrity over a whole lifetime of use. Of all the components present in the eye, none occupies more space than the vitreous. Little was known or written about its nature or function such that no earlier than a decade ago, people would debate its use, necessity, and role in retinal pathology. The fact that eyes function well without vitreous and our inability to visualize the vitreous and its interface with the retina until recently are largely responsible for our lack of understanding, but this is changing rapidly.

The vitreous cavity contains a physical transparent structure rather than only a liquid, suggesting usefulness and purpose for at least a portion of an eye's life cycle. Clearly, it can absorb a shock delivered to the globe, prevent complete collapse in the case of penetrating or perforating trauma, and constrain the advancement of certain infections such as fungi. With time, exposure to light, oxidative, metabolic, and mechanical stresses leads to the condensation of collagen fibers, liquefaction, and collapse of the vitreous body. The vitreous separates from its insertion onto the retina, starting a new phase of its career, allowing increased oxygenation to the retina and less structural support. This process of vitreolysis and posterior vitreous detachment is a slow process taking years to evolve. During this time, vitreomacular and vitreoretinal traction can lead to pathological changes sometimes with dire consequences for vision and the integrity of the retina. We are just discovering the full scope of these tractional pathologies. Indeed it is only in 2011 that the international classification of diseases (ICD) recognized vitreomacular traction as a separate entity with its own code. Such increased awareness of disease is not possible without considerable research. Indeed, our understanding of the biochemistry, physiology, and aging of normal vitreous has allowed us to better comprehend the steps leading to pathologic states. Strides made in the noninvasive imaging of ocular tissue have allowed us to visualize the consequences of vitreo-macular traction and follow it over time. Therapeutic strategies are being developed.

Despite all this activity, no book or monograph has ever been written on the vitreo-macular interface (VMI). Such a void needed to be filled. At the outset, we wanted to credit visionaries who studied the vitreous when no one else showed interest and provide current and future researchers with a valuable reference on VMI. This book begins with the anatomy, physiology, and aging changes of the interface. We look into the pathologic implications of anomalous adherences, its clinical manifestations, and report on the prevalence and incidence of various pathologic states. No book on the subject would be complete without due attention to imaging and its challenges and in particular possible venues to improve our ability to visualize and understand the vitreo-macular interface. Treatment strategies are appearing, even nonsurgical approaches. We gave ample space to report on achievements on the various venues imagined and explored to solve the adhesion using a nonsurgical approach. All known approaches whether successful, promising, or abandoned have been considered. Next, the challenges faced by clinical trials in this field are outlined so that future research can be facilitated. Finally, we consider what we have learned so far and how it can be applied to improve our future diagnostic and therapeutic abilities.

It is our hope that this book will be of use to all those fascinated, as we are, by the vitreo-macular interface—the basic scientist seeking to understand the intricacies of a barely visible tissue, the clinician faced with the challenges of patients whose VMI traction may lead to vision loss, imaging engineers, pharmacologists, and chemists. We hope to have sparked a better understanding and a foundation for future research.

<table>
<tr><td>Leuven, Belgium</td><td>Aniz Girach, MD</td></tr>
<tr><td>Lausanne, Switzerland</td><td>Marc D. de Smet, MDCM, PhD, FRCSC</td></tr>
</table>

Contents

Introduction: Unmet Medical Need

Colin A. McCannel and Donald S. Fong

1.1 Potential Diseases

1.1.1 "Classic" Vitreo-macular Traction Disease

Over the past two to three decades, understanding of the vitreoretinal interface's contribution to macular and retinal disease has immensely increased. The description of vitreo-macular traction syndrome dates back several decades (Reese et al. 1967, 1970). However, not until the advent of vitrectomy surgery and an expanding understanding of vitreo-macular traction disease pathophysiology have successful treatments been developed. Initially, vitrectomy surgery was proposed for pathologic changes involving incomplete separation of the vitreous or what today might be considered a typical vitreo-macular

traction syndrome (Smiddy et al. 1988; Margherio et al. 1989). While development of macular holes was first attributed to vitreo-macular traction (Gass 1988; Johnson and Gass 1988) during the evolution of the posterior vitreous detachment, the idea that relief of such vitreo-macular traction may facilitate closure of already present macular holes was not proposed until several years later (Kelly and Wendel 1991). Currently, there is thinking that vitreoretinal traction is as a contributory pathophysiologic component to diseases (e.g., diabetic macular edema) that were thought to have other mechanisms (Lewis et al. 1992).

With the use of optical coherence tomography imaging, the understanding of vitreoretinal traction in disease pathophysiology has expanded even more. Subtle degrees of vitreoretinal traction previously not visible could be recognized as causative or contributory to the formation of macular edema. Entirely new diseases are now recognized, such as myopic maculoschisis, principally caused by diffuse vitreo-macular traction (Takano and Kishi 1999; Akiba et al. 2000).

All of these conditions can be thought of as caused by a pathologic vitreoretinal separation, or lack thereof. Some of these conditions are successfully treated with vitrectomy surgery, with its inherent cost and morbidity. Other conditions, such as myopic maculoschisis, have been met with optimistic but inconsistent results following vitrectomy surgery (Kanda et al. 2003; Kwok et al. 2005; Hirakata and Hida 2006).

C.A. McCannel, MD, FACS (✉)
Vitreoretinal Surgeon, Kaiser Permanente Medical Center, Baldwin Park, CA, USA

Diabetic Retinopathy Photograph Reading Center, Regional Offices, Pasadena, CA, USA

Associate Clinical Professor of Ophthalmology, UCLA Medical School, Los Angeles, CA, USA
e-mail: cmccannel@jsei.ucla.edu

D.S. Fong, MD, MPH
Clinical Trials Research and DRS Reading Center, Kaiser Permanente Southern California, 100 S. Los Robles, Pasadena, CA 91101, USA
e-mail: donald.s.fong@kp.org

A. Girach, M.D. de Smet (eds.), *Diseases of the Vitreo-Macular Interface*, Essentials in Ophthalmology, DOI 10.1007/978-3-642-40034-6_1, © Springer-Verlag Berlin Heidelberg 2014

1.1.2 Diseases of Possible but Unproven Vitreoretinal Traction

There are additional diseases that may benefit from vitreoretinal separation should current speculation of the pathophysiology be proven correct. An increasing amount of consideration has been directed at whether exudative age-related macular degeneration and pigment epithelial detachments may be facilitated by macular vitreoretinal traction. It has been reported that a higher rate of incomplete vitreous detachment exists in eyes with AMD compared to non-AMD eyes (Weber-Krause and Eckardt 1996). Additional studies have similarly found an association between incomplete or absent posterior vitreous detachment and AMD in the elderly (Ondes et al. 2000; Krebs et al. 2007; Mojana et al. 2008; Lee et al. 2009). Whether the association represents a cause and effect relationship remains unproven. However, there is evidence that mechanical stress from traction on the retinal pigment epithelium may stimulate continued release of VEGF resulting in the development of exudative AMD (Seko et al. 1999).

1.1.3 Vitreoretinal Separation as Disease Prophylaxis?

With increasing understanding, vitreoretinal separation might also aid in the prevention of complications of diabetic retinopathy and rhegmatogenous complications of clear lens extractions. In the past, prophylactic posterior vitreous detachment was considered to help prevent complications of diabetic retinopathy (Ochoa-Contreras et al. 2000). To date, there is no proven benefit. A safe method of inducing a vitreous detachment may help in preventing complications of diabetic retinopathy, such as macular edema or proliferative disease.

A potential application for vitreoretinal interface cleaving may be clear lens extraction for treatment of myopia and presbyopia. Currently, clear lens extraction to correct myopia or presbyopia with multifocal intraocular lens placement has been associated with risk of rhegmatogenous retinal detachment (Colin et al. 1999; Kubaloğlu et al. 2004; Arne 2004). Pathologic or premature vitreous detachment that follows clear lens extraction leads to the retinal tears and detachments. Managing the vitreous detachment prior to clear lens extraction may render myopia or presbyopia correcting lenticular surgery a safer treatment option.

1.1.4 Summary

All of the aforementioned conditions and treatment approaches benefit from safe, atraumatic vitreous separation. While retina surgeons already have the surgical tools to separate the vitreous intraoperatively, approaches with less morbidity, complexity, and cost are desirable.

1.2 Frequency of Disease

Conditions known to benefit from vitreoretinal separation are common in most retina practices. Idiopathic macular holes occur at an age- and sex-adjusted incidence in 7.8 persons and 8.69 eyes per 100,000 population per year (McCannel et al. 2009). With a US population of approximately 309 million in 2010, that would amount to over 24,000 new macular holes in the United States annually. Rates of milder vitreo-macular traction disease are likely much higher. To date there is little knowledge of the actual incidence or prevalence of milder forms of vitreo-macular traction disease. Whether or not intervention for the various degrees of vitreo-macular traction disease is employed usually depends on the degree of vision compromise or natural history.

Myopia is quite common in the United States and Asia (Vitale et al. 2009; Pi et al. 2010). While myopic maculoschisis is uncommon or rare, the results of vitrectomy for treatment of this condition have been somewhat inconsistent. Once an alternative, safer approach for releasing the vitreo-macular traction is found, treatment of this condition might increase.

The prevalence of diabetes in the United States is increasing. In 1998, approximately 10.4 million persons carried a diagnosis of diabetes. Of those, greater than 90 % were afflicted with type II diabetes, a disease that is increasing in prevalence (Harris et al. 1998; Harris 2004). The rate and severity of retinopathy is affected greatly by duration and control of diabetes. Nonetheless, the prevalence of macular edema is estimated to be approximately 20 %, or approximately 2 million individuals. Currently, there is mounting evidence that vitreoretinal traction contributes to worsening of diabetic macular edema.

It has been estimated that by the year 2020, approximately three million Americans will suffer from age-related macular degeneration (AMD) and its vision loss complications (Friedman et al. 2004). If current speculations are correct and vitreoretinal traction is proven to contribute to the pathophysiology of AMD, pharmacologic vitreoretinal separation could become an important treatment adjunct in this condition.

Separation of the vitreoretinal interface in otherwise normal presbyopic or myopic eyes has the potential to reduce the risk of rhegmatogenous complications following lenticular refractive surgery. If this were the case, a tremendous number of individuals may benefit from additional options for managing presbyopia and myopia. According to the national census bureau, in 2010 over 100 million Americans were between the ages of 40 and 64 years old (www.census.gov 2012), what might be considered the pre-cataract surgery presbyopic age range. Myopes comprise a large portion of the Unites States population, over 40 % of individuals between the ages of 12 and 54 by some estimates (Vitale et al. 2009).

1.3 Current Treatments of Vitreoretinal Traction Disease

The current approach to treating diseases of the vitreoretinal interface is to perform a vitrectomy surgery when the severity of vision loss justifies the surgical risk.

1.3.1 Cost and Morbidity Considerations

Along with somewhat imperfect and sometimes disappointing outcomes, treatments are "invasive" and have risks and costs. Recognized risks of vitrectomy surgery include endophthalmitis, retinal detachment, and cataract formation, among others. From a patient perspective, a less invasive intervention with fewer risks and morbidity would be preferable. From a payer's perspective, spending fewer health care dollars on treatments that can accomplish the same, or better, is desirable. Lastly, from a societal perspective, treatments with lower risk, lower morbidity, and lower cost while maintaining excellent vision outcomes would improve patient and family cost and inconvenience. As such, medical therapies have generally evolved from complex, high risk, and high morbidity to less complex, lower risk, and lower morbidity. This has already occurred to some extent with the advent of small-gauge transconjunctival vitrectomy surgery. Transconjunctival vitrectomy surgeries consume less time and offer greater patient comfort and, debatably, better or at least earlier vision recovery. Another example is macular translocation surgery. In its prime, translocation surgery offered in some situations the best vision recovery and maintenance potential for exudative age-related macular degeneration but was rapidly eclipsed by anti-vascular endothelial growth factor therapy due to the far lesser risk and complexity of intravitreal injection. Intravitreal injections of antiangiogenic medications offer consistently better results than the complex and high-risk surgical intervention of macular translocation surgery.

1.3.2 Shortfalls of Current Treatments

Since it is common and appropriate to wait until the vision loss justifies the risk of intervention, many patients are left with improved vision, but not excellent vision. For example, patients diagnosed with vitreofoveal traction, or stage 1 macular holes, are appropriately not usually treated.

Approximately 50 % of such eyes will undergo spontaneous vitreous separation without macular hole formation and will maintain excellent vision. The other 50 % of eyes will suffer vision loss from progression to a stage 2 full thickness macular hole that requires surgical intervention for successful treatment. Despite excellent success rates of macular hole closure and vision recovery when surgery is ultimately performed, visual acuity does not often recover to the pre-macular hole level, and vision degrading distortion often persists. This example suggests that there is tremendous opportunity to refine our current approaches and outcomes.

1.4 Metrics to Evaluate New Treatment Options

Assessing new therapies involves rigorous and sound scientific study. In ophthalmologic disease, the principal outcome measure must be related to vision and usually is the measured visual acuity. Functional measures such as vision-related quality of life can additionally measure the overall impact of vision change on individuals' quality of life.

1.4.1 Visual Acuity

For new treatments, visual acuity should be investigated as the average visual acuity improvement or loss by person or as a percent of the population that either improves or worsens. For visual acuity change, the commonly accepted relevant outcome is a 3-line change on the ETDRS chart. This level of change is thought to be clinically meaningful. This is because a 3-line change (≥ 15 letters on the ETDRS chart) represents a doubling or halving of the visual angle. Investigators have shown that this level of change correlates with demonstrable differences in quality of life as measured with vision function questionnaires (Lindblad and Clemons 2005; Berdeaux et al. 2005; Finger et al 2008).

For treatments that are intended to replace or supplement existing treatments with already good outcomes, the investigation should assess whether the new treatment is non-inferior to the existing one. Should a new procedure or treatment be shown to achieve equivalent visual acuity or vision outcomes, then the new treatment's risk, morbidity, or expense may determine whether it gains traction among physicians and patients. However, non-inferiority trials, intended to demonstrate equivalence of treatments, are challenging to design and execute and their power limited at realistic sample sizes of such studies (Snapinn 2000; Wang and Hung 2003).

An example of a treatment that produces similar outcomes but at possibly lesser risk, or expense, might be macular hole treatment accomplished by injection of a pharmacologic agent instead of vitrectomy surgery followed by face down positioning. Even if the vision outcomes are similar, the injections might be preferable due to lower risk, morbidity, or expense.

Finally, for a treatment or intervention that is intended to alter the natural history of disease progression, there might not be changes in visual acuity. For example, if a stage I macular hole can be prevented from progressing to a full thickness macular hole, a therapeutic benefit would not be shown by improved visual acuity following intervention, but instead by lack of vision loss in comparison to the natural history. In the case of a stage I macular hole, the time course may be favorable for study, as macular hole progression often occurs in a limited period of time. On the other hand, studying an intervention intended to prevent vision loss from progressive myopic macular schisis, then the slow rate of disease progression would make such a study difficult to execute in a meaningful time frame. For such conditions, markers of success of the intervention other than visual acuity might be needed as clinical study outcome measures.

1.4.2 Nonvisual Acuity Assessments

When visual acuity is not a good outcome measure, anatomic and physiologic assessments may be used. Currently, the best method for evaluating vitreoretinal traction disease is optical coherence tomography (OCT). Specific measures include central retinal thickness, foveal thickness, and observable vitreoretinal traction associated with measures of macular thickness. The automated analysis provided by most OCT machines is helpful, but inaccuracies in the segmentation of the tissue planes are common and require manual confirmation of thickness measurements (Pierro et al. 2010; DRCR.net et al. 2007). Additionally, there are variations based on race, age, and gender that must be accounted for when using macular measurements (Kashani et al. 2010).

Judging whether or not vitreo-macular traction is present is inherently subjective. Agreed upon classification systems must be developed and utilized to minimize the subjectivity and allow for consistent grading of vitreo-macular traction severity. In the example of myopic retinoschisis, the anatomic documentation of the collapse of the schisis cavity while maintaining visual acuity might be considered a treatment success.

1.4.3 Safety

For vitreoretinal traction diseases that already have successful treatments, a new treatment must deliver at least similar vision-related outcomes and must be equally safe or safer. For conditions that currently do not have an excellent treatment, a new therapy must offer better outcomes than the natural history or current interventions. With regard to using the new treatment as a prophylaxis against the development of retinal disease, in the case of proliferative diabetic retinopathy or as prophylaxes against the development of known complications of procedures, such as retinal detachment following clear lens extraction, the new treatment must demonstrate an overall superb safety profile. In assessing safety, anatomic assessment is essential and must involve examination for retinal tears and detachment and possibly electroretinography and visual field testing to rule out retinal toxicity.

1.5 Profile of a Desired Product

An optimal therapy for disease with pathophysiologic contribution from vitreoretinal adhesions, or abnormal vitreoretinal interface, would be a treatment that safely separates vitreoretinal adhesions, both normal and abnormal. The release of the vitreoretinal traction must have a low morbidity and lower cost to patients and society than current management options while having a high efficacy. Additionally, controlled vitreous separation would allow treatment in situations in which the current therapeutic approach may not be available, is often deferred, or is considered too high risk.

> **Conclusion**
> Pharmacologic agents that effectively and safely lyse the vitreoretinal interface and adhesions have enormous potential for changing current practice by allowing not just treatment and earlier intervention of vitreoretinal interface disease but also conceivably offer prophylaxis or risk reduction.

Compliance with Ethical Requirements Dr Fong is a consultant for ThromboGenics and Allergan and receives grant support from Allergan. Dr McCannell has no conflicts of interest. No animal or human studies were carried out by the authors for this article.

References

Akiba J, Konno S, Sato E et al (2000) Retinal detachment and retinoschisis detected by optical coherence tomography in a myopic eye with a macular hole. Ophthalmic Surg Lasers 31(3):240–242

Arne JL (2004) Phakic intraocular lens implantation versus clear lens extraction in highly myopic eyes of 30- to 50-year-old patients. J Cataract Refract Surg 30(10):2092–2096

Berdeaux GH, Nordmann JP, Colin E et al (2005) Vision-related quality of life in patients suffering from age-related macular degeneration. Am J Ophthalmol 139:271–279

Colin J, Robinet A, Cochener B (1999) Retinal detachment after clear lens extraction for high myopia: seven-year follow-up. Ophthalmology 106(12):2281–2284

Diabetic Retinopathy Clinical Research Network, Krzystolik MG, Strauber SF et al (2007) Reproducibility of macular thickness and volume using Zeiss optical coherence tomography in patients with diabetic macular edema. Ophthalmology 114(8):1520–1525

Finger RP, Fleckenstein M, Holz FG et al (2008) Quality of life in age-related macular degeneration: a review of available vision-specific psychometric tools. Qual Life Res 17(4):559–574

Friedman DS, O'Colmain BJ, Munoz B et al (2004) Prevalence of age-related macular degeneration in the United States. Arch Ophthalmol 122:564–572

Gass JD (1988) Idiopathic senile macular hole. Its early stages and pathogenesis. Arch Ophthalmol 106(5): 629–639

Harris MI (2004) Diabetes in America: epidemiology and scope of the problem. Diabetes Care 21(Suppl 3): C11–C14

Harris MI, Flegal KM, Cowie CC et al (1998) Prevalence of diabetes, impaired fasting glucose, and impaired glucose tolerance in U.S. adults. The Third National Health and Nutrition Examination Survey, 1988–1994. Diabetes Care 21(4):518–524

Hirakata A, Hida T (2006) Vitrectomy for myopic posterior retinoschisis or foveal detachment. Jpn J Ophthalmol 50(1):53–61

http://www.census.gov/popest/data/intercensal/national/nat2010.html. Accessed April 23, 2012

Johnson RN, Gass JD (1988) Idiopathic macular holes. Observations, stages of formation, and implications for surgical intervention. Ophthalmology 95(7):917–924

Kanda S, Uemura A, Sakamoto Y, Kita H (2003) Vitrectomy with internal limiting membrane peeling for macular retinoschisis and retinal detachment without macular hole in highly myopic eyes. Am J Ophthalmol 136(1):177–180

Kashani AH, Zimmer-Galler IE, Shah SM et al (2010) Retinal thickness analysis by race, gender, and age using Stratus OCT. Am J Ophthalmol 149(3):496–502

Kelly NE, Wendel RT (1991) Vitreous surgery for idiopathic macular holes. Results of a pilot study. Arch Ophthalmol 109(5):654–659

Krebs I, Brannath W, Glittenberg C et al (2007) Posterior vitreomacular adhesion: a potential risk factor for exudative age-related macular degeneration? Am J Ophthalmol 144:741–746

Kubaloğlu A, Yazicioğlu T, Tacer S (2004) Small incision clear lens extraction for correction of high myopia. Eur J Ophthalmol 14(1):1–6

Kwok AK, Lai TY, Yip WW (2005) Vitrectomy and gas tamponade without internal limiting membrane peeling for myopic foveoschisis. Br J Ophthalmol 89(9):1180–1183

Lee SJ, Lee CS, Koh HJ (2009) Posterior vitreomacular adhesion and risk of exudative age related macular degeneration: Paired eye study. Am J Ophthalmol 147:621–626

Lewis H, Abrams GW, Blumenkranz MS et al (1992) Vitrectomy for diabetic macular traction and edema associated with posterior hyaloidal traction. Ophthalmology 99(5):753–759

Lindblad AS, Clemons TE (2005) Responsiveness of the National Eye Institute Visual Function Questionnaire to progression to advanced age-related macular degeneration, vision loss, and lens opacity: AREDS Report No. 14. Arch Ophthalmol 123:1207–1214

Margherio RR, Trese MT, Margherio AR et al (1989) Surgical management of vitreomacular traction syndromes. Ophthalmology 96(9):1437–1445

McCannel CA, Ensminger JL, Diehl NN et al (2009) Population-based incidence of macular holes. Ophthalmology 116(7):1366–1369

Mojana F, Cheng L, Bartsch DG et al (2008) The role of abnormal vitreomacular adhesion in age-related macular degeneration: Spectral optical coherence tomography and surgical results. Am J Ophthalmol 146:218–227

Ochoa-Contreras D, Delsol-Coronado L, Buitrago ME et al (2000) Induced posterior vitreous detachment by intravitreal sulfur hexafluoride (SF6) injection in patients with nonproliferative diabetic retinopathy. Acta Ophthalmol Scand 78(6):687–688

Ondes F, Yilmaz G, Acar MA et al (2000) Role of the vitreous in age-related macular degeneration. Jpn J Ophthalmol 44:91–93

Pi LH, Chen L, Liu Q et al (2010) Refractive status and prevalence of refractive errors in suburban school-age children. Int J Med Sci 7(6):342–353

Pierro L, Giatsidis SM, Mantovani E et al (2010) Macular thickness interoperator and intraoperator reproducibility in healthy eyes using 7 optical coherence tomography instruments. Am J Ophthalmol 150(2):199–204

Reese AB, Jones IS, Cooper WC (1967) Macular changes secondary to vitreous traction. Am J Ophthalmol 64(3):544–549

Reese AB, Jones IS, Cooper WC (1970) Vitreomacular traction syndrome confirmed histologically. Am J Ophthalmol 69(6):975–977

Seko Y, Seko Y, Fujikura H et al (1999) Induction of vascular endothelial growth factor after application of mechanical stress to retinal pigment epithelium of the rat in vitro. Invest Ophthalmol Vis Sci 40: 3287–3291

Smiddy WE, Michels RG, Glaser BM et al (1988) Vitrectomy for macular traction caused by incomplete vitreous separation. Arch Ophthalmol 106(5):624–628

Snapinn SM (2000) Noninferiority trials. Curr Control Trials Cardiovasc Med 1(1):19–21

Takano M, Kishi S (1999) Foveal retinoschisis and retinal detachment in severely myopic eyes with posterior staphyloma. Am J Ophthalmol 128(4):472–476

Vitale S, Sperduto RD, Ferris FL 3rd (2009) Increased prevalence of myopia in the United States between 1971–1972 and 1999–2004. Arch Ophthalmol 127(12):1632–1639

Wang SJ, Hung HM (2003) Assessing treatment efficacy in noninferiority trials. Control Clin Trials 24(2):147–155

Weber-Krause B, Eckardt U (1996) Häufigkeit einer hinteren Glaskörperabhebung bei Augen mit und ohne altersabhängige Makuladegeneration [Incidence of posterior vitreous detachment in eyes with and without age-related macular degeneration. An ultrasonic study]. Ophthalmologe 93:660–665

The Epidemiology of Vitreo-macular Interface Diseases

2

Andrew R.H. Simpson and Timothy L. Jackson

2.1 Introduction

Historically the vitreo-macular interface has been assessed by biomicroscopy. It is possible to determine the presence of an abnormal vitreo-macular interface by biomicroscopy alone, although due to the inherent difficulties of visually assessing the transparent vitreous, biomicroscopy has been shown to substantially underestimate the true extent to which abnormal vitreo-macular adhesion (VMA) exists. One such study by Gallemore et al. (2000) showed that vitreous adhesions were detected in 30 % of eyes with certain retinal diseases assessed by optical coherence tomography (OCT), compared with 8 % assessed by biomicroscopy alone. The widespread introduction of OCT over the last two decades has led to a significant advance in the understanding of the role of the vitreous in the pathogenesis of several retinal diseases.

The term VMA describes the anatomic state whereby the posterior vitreous face lies in apposition to the fovea, often with separation of the vitreous face from the surrounding macula. Therefore, VMA is a kind of incomplete poste-

rior vitreous detachment (PVD). VMA usually exists without causing any structural or functional abnormality. If, however, the tractional forces applied to the macula are significant, visual symptoms may develop, either through retinal disorders associated with VMA, such as idiopathic macular hole, or in isolation, where this is usually referred to as vitreo-macular traction (VMT) or VMT syndrome.

More recently, the term symptomatic VMA has been introduced to describe any form of VMA-causing symptoms. This encompasses VMT syndrome, macular hole (where there is persisting VMA), and other conditions where VMA may contribute to the pathogenesis or clinical course of an underlying disease, such as neovascular age-related macular degeneration (wet AMD) or diabetic macular edema (DME).

Of the conditions grouped together under the symptomatic VMA label, the quality and extent of the epidemiological data vary enormously. For macular hole, which has for a long time been associated with VMA, there is a large evidence base. For VMT there is very little evidence about incidence and prevalence. For DME and wet AMD, occurring in the context of VMA, there is a limited, but expanding evidence base. This chapter aims to survey the epidemiological data on symptomatic VMA. In addition, we attempted to estimate the total incidence and prevalence of symptomatic VMA using the data that were available.

A.R.H. Simpson, MBBS • T.L. Jackson, PhD,
FRCOphth (✉)
Department of Ophthalmology,
King's College London, King's College Hospital,
Denmark Hill, London, SE5 9RS, UK
e-mail: andy.simpson@doctors.org.uk;
t.jackson1@nhs.net

A. Girach, M.D. de Smet (eds.), *Diseases of the Vitreo-Macular Interface*, Essentials in Ophthalmology,
DOI 10.1007/978-3-642-40034-6_2, © Springer-Verlag Berlin Heidelberg 2014

2.2 Macular Hole

2.2.1 Vitreo-macular Adhesion and Macular Hole

Lister, back in 1924, first suspected that the vitreous influenced the development of macular holes (Lister 1924); however, it was much later that Gass, in the pre-OCT era, described how focal shrinkage of the vitreous at the fovea, with the resultant traction, led to macular hole formation (Johnson and Gass 1988; Gass 1988). His hypothesis has since been confirmed by numerous OCT studies (Hee et al. 1995; Gaudric et al. 1999; Chauhan et al. 2000; Tanner et al. 2001). He classified macular holes into 4 stages: stage 1, macular cyst; stage 2, small (<400 µm in diameter (Gass 1995)), full-thickness hole; stage 3, large (≥400 µm in diameter (Gass 1995)), full-thickness hole with vitreous attached; and stage 4, large hole with detached vitreous. Although the majority of macular holes begin with an abnormal interaction between the fovea and the posterior vitreous face, there is very little data that shows the rate that this interaction can be detected by OCT. Gallemore reported VMA rates in macular hole, as determined by OCT, to be 16 % (Gallemore et al. 2000), although as mentioned, this figure is likely to be a gross underestimation of the true rate of VMA in macular holes, possibly due to the limitations of OCT, especially time-domain models as used in this study, to detect the posterior vitreous face when it is in very close apposition to the macula.

2.2.2 Prevalence

A number of population-based studies have reported the prevalence of macular holes. The Beaver Dam Eye Study was a population-based study performed in Wisconsin, USA, beginning in 1987 (Klein et al. 1991). A total of 4,926 people between the age of 43 and 84 years old participated. As part of each participant's examination, stereoscopic and non-stereoscopic fundus color photographs of the optic disc and macular region were obtained for each eye. Fundus photographs were assessed in a masked fashion, with macular holes recorded as present if there was evidence of "sharply defined round or oval full-thickness holes involving the foveal area" (Klein et al. 1994).

The Beaver Dam Eye Study calculated that the prevalence of macular hole increased with age, with 0 cases per 1,000 population for people aged 43–54 years, 1.3/1,000 for those aged 55–64, 3.4/1,000 for those aged 64–74, and 3.8/1,000 for those aged 75 years and above. The overall rate in all patients was 1.4 cases per 1,000 (0.14 %). In addition, macular holes were reported more frequently in patients with coexisting epiretinal membranes (age-controlled odd ratio = 16.10, 95 % confidence interval (CI) 5.37–48.42).

The Blue Mountains Eye Study, a similar population-based study, was undertaken in Australia between 1992 and 1993 (Mitchell et al. 1997). Eighty-eight percent of the eligible population, aged 49 and over, underwent a detailed eye examination and fundus photography. Six out of 3,654 subjects (0.16 %) had a full-thickness macular hole.

The Baltimore Eye Study screened 5,300 subjects aged 40 years and older and reported 6 cases (0.11 %) of macular hole that were responsible for visual impairment, defined as vision worse than 20/40 and better than 20/200 in the better eye (Rahmani et al. 1996). It is important to note that because only eyes with vision worse than 20/40 were counted, macular holes that had no or minimal impact on vision were excluded; therefore 0.11 % is an underestimate of the true prevalence. This figure is however still useful when trying to determine the symptomatic burden of macular hole, and ultimately VMA, on the general population.

The prevalence of macular holes was also reported in the Beijing Eye Study (Wang et al. 2006). A total of 8,653 eyes of 4,346 subjects, aged 40 years and older, had fundus photographs suitable for assessment. Seven people (0.16 %) had a macular hole, which included 1 bilateral case.

Another large study compared rates between urban and rural populations in southern India (Sen et al. 2008). Thirteen subjects (2 bilateral cases) out of 7,774 (0.17 %) were diagnosed with macular holes, with a mean age of 67 years.

There was no difference in prevalence found between the urban and rural populations.

Taking these studies together, and weighted for the relative contribution of each based on study size, the average prevalence is 149 per 100,000 (Table 2.1).

2.2.3 Incidence

McCannel et al. are one of the only groups to have estimated the annual incidence of macular hole (McCannel et al. 2009). In a predominantly Caucasian population in the USA, idiopathic macular holes occurred at an age- and sex-adjusted rate of 7.8 persons (8.7 eyes) per 100,000 population per year. A follow-up to the Beaver Dam Eye Study reported a 10-year incidence of 0.7 % of the population (la Cour and Friis 2002), equating to approximately 30 cases per 100,000 annually. Combining these studies, weighted for study size, gives a mean incidence of 8.8 cases per 100,000 (Table 2.1).

2.2.4 Prevalence of Vision Loss

Idiopathic macular holes are predominantly unilateral; however the above population studies report an approximate 10 % rate of bilateral occurrence. The 6 macular holes reported in the Baltimore Eye Study represented 3.8 % of all cases of visual impairment (Rahmani et al. 1996). Similarly, the Beijing Eye Study reported that full-thickness macular holes accounted for 2 % of cases of visual impairment, defined as BCVA in the better eye worse than 20/60 and better or equal to 20/400, and no cases of blindness, defined as BCVA worse than 20/400 (Wang et al. 2006).

2.2.5 Burden of Disease

Hikichi et al. (1995) identified 154 macular holes and found that 26.0 % ($n = 40$) were classified stage 1 according to the Gass classification (Gass 1988), 16.2 % ($n = 25$) stage 2, 37.7 % ($n = 58$) stage 3, and 20.1 % ($n = 31$) stage 4. The combined proportion of stage 2 and 3 holes ($n = 83$), where

there is by definition VMA, is 72.8 %, compared to 27.2 % with stage 4 holes where there is no VMA. Stage 1 macular cysts can be excluded as they seldom cause significant visual symptoms. These figures can be used to estimate the burden of macular holes that can be attributed to VMA in the general population. The previously described population studies show a macular hole prevalence of approximately 0.11–0.17 % (as these figures are derived from diagnoses made primarily by fundus photography, they are not likely to include macular cysts as well), which suggests that 0.8–1.2 persons per 1,000 of the general population have a symptomatic macular hole with VMA. If we apply a similar calculation to the incidence rates available, then this suggests that between 5.7 and 21.8 people per 100,000 population per year in the USA could develop a macular hole secondary to VMA. These calculations may somewhat underestimate the true proportion of eyes in which VMA contributed to macular hole formation, as stage 3 holes may evolve to stage 4, and thereby be excluded from this analysis, even if VMA played a role in their pathogenesis.

2.3 Epiretinal Membrane

2.3.1 Vitreo-macular Adhesion and Epiretinal Membrane

In the seminal paper on the subject, Foos described how glial cells migrate to the surface of the internal limiting membrane (ILM), commonly after PVD, leading to ERM formation (Foos 1977). He also observed that if an ERM formed before a PVD developed, a vitreous layer may be present underneath the ERM. Epiretinal membranes are classically described as being associated with PVD (Wise 1975; Wiznia 1986; Hirokawa et al. 1986; Appiah et al. 1988; Sidd et al. 1982) rather than VMA.

The nature of any association between VMA and ERM is somewhat uncertain. Unlike macular hole, where there is compelling evidence that VMA plays an important if not primary role in its pathogenesis, ERMs often occur in complete absence of VMA, as might occur following pars plana vitrectomy for retinal detachment.

Table 2.1 Summary of Studies Included for Calculation of Prevalence and Incidence

Condition	Study	Age range (years)	Study size (n)	Prevalence (per 100,000 population)	Annual incidence (per 100,000 population)[a]
Macular hole	Beaver Dam (Klein et al. 1994)	43–84	4,926	140	30 (la Cour and Friis 2002)
	Blue Mountains (Mitchell et al. 1997)	≥49	3,654	160	–
	Baltimore (Rahmani et al. 1996)	≥40	5,300	110	–
	Beijing (Wang et al. 2006)	≥40	4,346	160	–
	Sen et al. (2008)	–	7,774	170	–
	McCannel et al. (2009)	47.5–89.6	106,470	NA	7.8
	Weighted average, range, or total[b]	≥43	26,000	149	8.8
ERM	Beaver Dam (Klein et al. 1994)	43–84	4,802	11,800	–
	Blue Mountain (Mitchell et al. 1997)	≥49	3,654	6,700	–
	Jackson et al. (2013)	16.1–93.5	8,257	NA	3.2[c]
	Weighted average, range or total[b]	≥16.1	8,456	9,600	3.2
VMT syndrome	Jackson et al. (2013)	32.4–89.2	8,257	22.5[c]	0.56[c]
	Weighted average, range or total[b]	32.4–89.2	8,257	22.5	0.56
Wet AMD	The Eye Diseases Prevalence Research Group (Friedman et al. 2004)	≥40	Pooled population studies	1,020	NA
	Beaver Dam (Klein et al. 2002)	43–86	2,764	–	90
	Blue Mountains (Wang et al. 2007)	≥49	1,952	–	3,70[d]
	Rotterdam (Klaver et al. 2001)	≥55	4,953	–	80
	Miyazaki et al. (2005)	≥50	961	NA	160
	Weighted average range or total[b]	–	–	1,020	143
DME	Minassian et al. (2012)	–	–	320	–
	Weighted average, range or total[b]	–	–	320	–

AMD age-related macular degeneration, *DME* diabetic macular edema, *ERM* epiretinal membrane, *VMT* vitreo-macular traction

[a]Incidence rates were calculated on an annual basis, although several of the studies reported their results over longer time periods

[b]The weighted average was the mean incidence or prevalence of all groups combined, adjusted for the size of each study, such that larger studies had a proportionally greater impact on the final average than smaller studies

[c]Only includes cases that underwent vitrectomy

[d]Includes cases of significant geographic atrophy

A significant minority of ERMs may however be associated with VMA or VMT. Hirokawa et al. reviewed 250 cases of idiopathic ERMs and reported that 39 (15.6 %) cases had partial PVD with either VMA (10 eyes, 4.0 %) or VMT (29 eyes, 11.6 %), with complete PVD present in 155 (62.0 %) cases (Hirokawa et al. 1986). A similar study by Appiah et al. reported 10.9 % (43/395) of ERMs were associated with partial PVD and VMA (Appiah et al. 1988).

2.3.2 Prevalence

In the Beaver Dam Eye Study (Klein et al. 1994), an ERM was present in at least one eye of 11.8 % (565/4,802) of the population, where at least one eye could be graded, and present in both eyes of 2.4 % (110/4,639). There was a strong link to prevalence of ERM and increasing age, although unlike macular hole, there was no difference found between genders. This study, performed in the late 1980s, estimated that a total of 30 million people aged 43–86 years had an ERM in at least one eye in the USA.

The next population-based study to report the prevalence of ERM was the Blue Mountains Eye Study, where ERM presence was assessed both clinically and from fundus photographs (Mitchell et al. 1997). ERMs were observed in 317 eyes of 243 subjects, giving an overall prevalence of ERM in at least one eye of 6.7 % (243/3,654). Seventy-four subjects (31 %) had bilateral ERMs. There was a strong link with increasing age: 1.9 % in people aged less than 60 years, 7.2 % in people aged 60–69 years, 11.6 % in people aged 70–79 years, and 9.3 % in people aged 80 years and over.

The weighted-average prevalence of ERM in these population studies was 9,600 per 100,000 (Table 2.1).

2.3.3 Incidence

There are no studies that specifically investigated the incidence of ERM. Jackson et al. undertook a national database study of the surgical case mix in 31 vitreoretinal units in the United Kingdom over an 8-year period (Jackson et al. 2013). They reported that 995 of 8,257 (12.1 %) pars plana vitrectomies were for ERM. There were approximately 16,500 pars plana vitrectomies undertaken in a 1-year period (2009–2010) in the United Kingdom (Hospital Episode Statistics 2012), and therefore the annual incidence of ERM undergoing surgery is estimated at 3.2 per 100,000 population, calculated from the 2010 population estimate of 62.3 million (Office for National Statistics 2011).

2.3.4 Burden of Disease

Using the data from the above studies, weighted for their size, such that larger studies contribute proportionally more to the final aggregate mean, it is possible to make an approximate estimation of the number of people with ERM associated with VMA or VMT. The weighted-mean ERM prevalence from the Beaver Dam Eye Study and Blue Mountains Eye Study is 9.6 %, and the weighted-mean rate of VMA/VMT in ERM (estimated from Hirokawa et al. (1986) and Appiah et al. (1988)) is 12.7 %. These figures, combined, equate to a VMA/ERM prevalence of 1.2 %, with approximately 1.2 million people affected in the USA (calculated from 2010 population estimate of 99.0 million people aged 50 years and over (The 2012 Statistical Abstract 2012)) and 2.2 million people affected in the European Union (calculated from 2010 population estimate of 182.9 million people aged 50 years and over (European Population Statistics 2012)). This may underestimate the total number affected assuming some people aged less than 50 years will also have ERM with either VMA or VMT. Conversely, many of these cases may be asymptomatic, and the proportion with symptomatic VMA is not known. In this respect the incidence figure, based on Jackson et al.'s database study(Jackson et al. 2013), may be more representative of the burden of symptomatic VMA, as all cases underwent surgery. That study may however underestimate the true incidence, assuming not all people with symptomatic ERM will have surgery.

2.4 Vitreo-macular Traction Syndrome

2.4.1 Vitreo-macular Adhesion and Vitreo-macular Traction Syndrome

Vitreo-macular traction syndrome is, by definition, a disease caused by abnormal VMA. In 1967, Reese et al. first described VMT syndrome as a condition where "vitreous detachment exerts a pull on the macula through a vitreo-macular adhesion," with subsequent macular and submacular edema and at later stages retinal cystic changes (Reese et al. 1967). He postulated that the edema was caused by a combination of the hydraulic effect of the traction and macular ischemia, because the macula was separated from its choroidal blood supply. A few years later he confirmed his findings histologically (Reese et al. 1970).

2.4.2 Incidence and Prevalence

There are limited epidemiological data available for VMT syndrome. There have been no population studies that have reported the prevalence or incidence of the disease. There have been a few case series, mostly surgical, which provide basic demographic data (Smiddy et al. 1988; Margherio et al. 1989; McDonald et al. 1994; Melberg et al. 1995). By far the largest case series was performed by Margherio et al. with a total of 106 patients deemed high risk for macular hole due to vitreo-macular traction, who went on to have a vitrectomy (Margherio et al. 1989). The mean age of patient was 67 years, with a female preponderance of 62 % ($n=66$). The other much smaller case series reported similar demographics.

A similar calculation to the one that we described above, in the ERM section, was performed to estimate the incidence of VMT undergoing vitrectomy, using Jackson et al.'s national database study (Jackson et al. 2013). A total of 171 out of 8,257 (2.1 %) vitrectomies were undertaken for VMT. The annual incidence of VMT undergoing surgery is therefore estimated at 0.56 per 100,000 population in the United Kingdom.

In the absence of any reported prevalence figures for VMT, it is possible to make a very approximate estimate of prevalence, based on the relative proportion of VMT and macular holes undergoing surgery. Of the 8,257 vitrectomies in Jackson's study, VMT accounted for 171 cases, and macular hole 1,131 (Jackson et al. 2013). If the prevalence figures are similar, then VMT would have a prevalence that is 15.1 % of that of macular hole, or 22.5 cases per 100,000 people. This figure may underestimate the true prevalence of VMT, as VMT may be less likely to progress to surgery than macular hole.

2.4.3 Burden of Disease

All cases of VMT can be considered to have symptomatic VMA – in many respects VMT syndrome is the purest form of symptomatic VMA. Therefore the estimated incidence of VMT given above can be considered the burden of surgical disease. This most likely underestimates the true incidence of VMT, as not all cases with VMT undergo surgery.

In a study of ocriplasmin for VMT (personal correspondence L. Bouckaert, data on file, ThromboGenics, Leuven, Belgium), 19 % (15/78) of cases in the placebo arm ultimately required surgery, despite the trial selectively recruiting patients in whom vitrectomy was originally intended. If we assume that the number of cases proceeding to surgery is therefore only 19 % of those presenting to vitreoretinal surgeons, then the incidence of VMT increases from 0.56 per 100,000 per year to 2.95. This may overestimate the incidence of VMT as some of the cases in the ocriplasmin trial may subsequently have undergone surgery, but conversely there is likely to be a substantial proportion of patients who have VMT but do not present to a vitreoretinal surgeon and elect to undergo surgery.

2.5 Neovascular Age-Related Macular Degeneration

2.5.1 Age-Related Macular Degeneration and Vitreo-macular Adhesion

Over the last decade, evidence is emerging that the vitreo-macular interface influences the pathogenesis and clinical course of wet AMD (Simpson et al. 2012). A systematic review and meta-analysis by ourselves (Jackson et al. 2012) investigated the association of VMA and AMD. In neovascular AMD, the prevalence of VMA and PVD were 17 % (904 eyes) and 41 % (251 eyes), respectively. The prevalence of VMA was 2.17 times that of controls and 2.54 times that of dry AMD. The prevalence of PVD was lower than controls (relative risk = 0.79) and dry AMD (relative risk = 0.56). These data suggest that VMA is associated with wet AMD, although they do not necessarily establish a causative link.

2.5.2 Prevalence

Age-related macular degeneration is the leading cause of irreversible blindness in the developed world (Sommer et al. 1991; Klein et al. 1991; Klaver et al. 1998; Wang et al. 2000; Munoz et al. 2000; Weih et al. 2000). The Eye Diseases Prevalence Research Group conducted a large pooled analysis from the main population-based studies to attempt to identify the prevalence of AMD (Friedman et al. 2004). The overall prevalence of neovascular AMD and/or geographic atrophy was estimated to be 1.47 % (95 % CI 1.38–1.55 %). When applying age-, gender- and race-/ethnicity-specific rates to different populations around the world, the USA, Western Europe, and Australia are estimated to have 1.75 million, 3.35 million, and 130,000 individuals affected by AMD, respectively. The data for neovascular AMD alone showed a prevalence of 1.02 % (95 % CI 0.93–1.11), with an estimated 1.22 million cases in the USA. With an ever-growing and ageing worldwide population, these figures will increase substantially over the next few decades (Friedman et al. 2004).

2.5.3 Prevalence of Vision Loss

AMD causes significant visual disability. The Salisbury Eye Evaluation Study in the USA randomly sampled patients aged 65–84 years (Munoz et al. 2000). Out of the 2,520 subjects examined, 85 (3.8 %) were visually impaired (better eye worse than 20/40 and better than 20/200) and 21 (0.8 %) were classified as blind (better eye worse than 20/200). Nine of the 21 (43 %) bilaterally blind cases and 17 of the 85 (20 %) visual impairment cases were due to AMD (dry or wet not distinguished). In the United Kingdom, a total of 13,788 persons were registered blind between April 1999 and March 2000 (Bunce and Wormald 2008). Age-related macular degeneration accounted for 7,881 (57.2 %) of all cases and was the leading cause of blind registrations in patients aged 65 years and over.

2.5.4 Incidence

The Beaver Dam Eye Study reported 5-year and 10-year incidence rates of neovascular AMD of 1.8 and 4.1 %, respectively, in individuals aged 75 years and older (Klein et al. 1997; Klein et al. 2002). Similarly, The Blue Mountains Eye Study reported 5-year and 10-year incidence of "late AMD" (defined as neovascular AMD or geographic atrophy) of 1.1 and 3.7 %, respectively, although these figures include all the study's age groups (≥49 years) (Mitchell et al. 2002; Wang et al. 2007). The Rotterdam Eye Study was a large population-based study of people aged 55 years and older (Klaver et al. 2001). A total of 4,953 people were assessed at baseline and 2 years to determine 2-year incidence rates of both neovascular and atrophic AMD. Twelve subjects developed AMD over this period, with neovascular AMD accounting for eight of these cases. The overall incidence rate for AMD was 1.2 cases per

1,000 people per year and 0.8 cases of neovascular AMD per 1,000 per year. The cumulative 2-year incidence of all subjects was 0.24 %, increasing to 1.75 % when considering only those aged 85 years and older.

The 5-year incidence of developing either neovascular AMD or geographic atrophy was 0.8 % in a Japanese population study aged over 50 years (Miyazaki et al. 2005). Incidence rates of neovascular AMD in the United Kingdom population, aged 50 years and older, are estimated at 2.3 per 1,000 women per year and 1.4 per 1,000 men per year (Owen et al. 2012). The same study estimated the total number of new cases of neovascular AMD in the United Kingdom per year to be approximately 39,800.

The overall weighted-average incidence across these studies was calculated at 143 per 100,000 per year (Table 2.1).

2.5.5 Burden of Disease

Based on the Eye Diseases Prevalence Research Group data presented above, it is estimated that the prevalence of wet AMD is 1,020 per 100,000. If 16.7 % of these eyes have VMA (Jackson et al. 2012), then the prevalence of AMD occurring with VMA is approximately 170.3 per 100,000. This may overestimate the true burden of disease, as 10.4 % of age-matched, healthy control eyes also have VMA (Jackson et al. 2012) and it is perhaps only the increase in VMA that is significant. Conversely, many more cases of VMA probably coexist with AMD, as VMA is only apparent on OCT if the vitreous is partially separated at the macula. Cases where the vitreous is fully attached are not usually visible using OCT, as the posterior hyaloid face lies in direct apposition to the ILM.

2.6 Diabetic Macular Edema

2.6.1 Diabetic Macular Edema and Vitreo-macular Adhesion

The primary pathogenic factor in DME is a microvasculopathy, although the vitreo-macular interface probably plays a role. In 1988, Nasrallah et al. demonstrated that patients with diabetic retinopathy and coexisting DME were less likely to have a PVD, compared with patients who did not have DME (20 % vs 55 %, respectively) (Nasrallah et al. 1988). Lewis et al. performed a small number of vitrectomies on eyes with coexistent DME and what was described at the time as a "thickened and taut premacular posterior hyaloid" (Lewis et al. 1992). Nine out of 10 eyes had an improvement in vision, and all showed a reduction in the edema. Since then, a number of studies have reported similar beneficial outcomes, both functionally and anatomically, following vitrectomy for the treatment of VMA and VMT (van Effenterre et al. 1993; Harbour et al. 1996; Pendergast 1998; Pendergast et al. 2000), although the evidence is not conclusive as there are also studies which show no improvement (Laidlaw 2008).

A systemic review and meta-analysis identified several clinical studies from which an estimate of the prevalence of VMT in DME was made (Jackson et al. 2012). Across seven studies, there were 548 eyes with DME in which the VMT status was known. The overall mean prevalence of VMT, weighted for study size, was 17 %. Most of the studies forming the meta-analysis were surgical in nature, and it is not certain that the results would be generalizable to a nonsurgical setting. It is interesting though that Gallemore reported a similar prevalence of 17 % (7 out of 42 eyes) of VMA/VMT in eyes with diabetic retinopathy (Gallemore et al. 2000).

2.6.2 Diabetic Retinopathy and Vitreo-macular Adhesion

It is likely that the vitreous plays a role in the development of proliferative diabetic retinopathy, as the vitreous provides a scaffold for new blood vessel growth and vitreous traction on new blood vessels at the disc or elsewhere may lead to vitreous hemorrhage (Davis and Blodi 2001). It is possible also that PVD alters the diffusion of proangiogenic factors and alters vitreous oxygenation, and this may influence the likelihood of developing neovascularization (Simpson et al. 2012). It is however very difficult to quantify these interactions, and since new vessel growth is not typically at the macula, it is considered outside the remit of this chapter on VMA. Of interest though, Jackson et al.'s database study found that 389 of 8,257 pars plana vitrectomies (4.7 %) were undertaken for diabetic eye disease with traction (Jackson et al. 2013). It is not known how many of these had macular involvement, but it is likely to be a very high proportion given that macular involvement is the usual indication for vitrectomy in this setting.

2.6.3 Prevalence

It is estimated that there are approximately 171 million cases of diabetes worldwide (Wild et al. 2004), with several studies predicting a large increase to as much as 366 million over the next two decades (Wild et al. 2004; King et al. 1998). The prevalence of diabetes worldwide has been estimated at 2.8 % in 2000 and predicted to increase to 4.4 % by the year 2030 (Wild et al. 2004).

Diabetic macular edema is a complication of both type 1 and 2 diabetes mellitus, in which a microvasculopathy leads to fluid leaking into the tissue of the macula. A large literature review estimated the prevalence of DME among people with diabetes to be in the range of 0.85–12.3 % (Chen et al. 2010) (equating to between 1.5 and 21.0 million people worldwide [calculated from 171 million total cases of diabetes (Wild et al. 2004)]), with the prevalence and incidence varying significantly depending on type of diabetes, duration of disease, and insulin dependence (Chen et al. 2010). A recent study in England (Minassian et al. 2012) estimated that, in 2010, 7.1 % of all diabetic patients had DME in one or both eyes, totalling approximately to 166,325 people. This is equivalent to 0.32 % of the whole population (population of England, 2010: estimated at 52.2 million (Office for National Statistics 2011)).

2.6.4 Prevalence of Vision Loss

Minassian et al. reported on the prevalence of visual impairment attributable to DME in the Welsh diabetic population who underwent retinopathy screening in 2004–2005 (Minassian et al. 2012). The prevalence of DME of any severity in one or both eyes, just one eye, or both eyes, was 7.05, 4.72, and 2.33 %, respectively. Visual loss attributable to DME in this diabetic population was as follows: 2.75 % had BCVA <20/20 in at least one eye, 2.64 % had BCVA between 20/20 and 20/200 in at least one eye, 0.23 % had BCVA between 20/63 and 20/200 in the better seeing eye, and 0.109 % had BCVA of less than or equal to 20/200 in both eyes. They estimated the health and social care direct costs of DME for 2010 in England to be £120 million (Minassian et al. 2012) (approximately $193 million US Dollars from May 2012 exchange rates).

2.6.5 Incidence

The Wisconsin Epidemiological Study of Diabetic Retinopathy (WESDR) was a large population-based study of type 1 and 2 diabetics (Klein et al. 1984). The 25-year cumulative incidence of DME and clinically significant DME (defined as presence of retinal thickening or hard exudates at or within 500 μm of the center of the macula) in 520 type 1 diabetic subjects was 29 and 17 %, respectively (Klein et al. 2009). At the time of their report (~2008) there were thought to be 515,000 to 1.3 million people in the USA with type 1 diabetes, and they therefore estimated that, over a 25-year period, 149,000–377,000 of these will develop DME and 88,000–221,000 will develop clinically significant DME.

A longitudinal study of diabetic patients undergoing retinopathy screening in the United Kingdom reported a 2-year incidence of clinically significant DME of 4.79 % (Ling et al. 2002). A Swedish study followed a group of 1,585 diabetics, both type 1 and 2, for 3 years and found an incidence of clinically significant DME of 2.3 % per year (Henricsson et al. 1999).

Interestingly, the annualized incidence of DME in the WESDR was lower in the last follow-up period (0.9 % between 1994–1999 and 2005–2007), compared to the previous 3 follow-up periods (2.3 % between 1980–1982 and 1984–1986, 2.1 % between 1984–1986 and 1990–1992, and 2.3 % between 1990–1992 and 1994–1996) (Klein et al. 2009). The authors suggested that this decline might be due to better glycemic control, as mean glycosylated hemoglobin A1 went from 10.7 % in the first period to 9.4 % in the fourth period. A Danish study also reported a decline in DME rates over time (Rossing 2005).

2.6.6 Burden of Disease

Unlike the studies of VMA and AMD, the studies of DME were principally describing pathological VMT, and hence all may be considered to be clinically significant. Based on a prevalence of DME of 7.1 % (Minassian et al. 2012) and 17 % prevalence of coexisting VMT, the total burden of disease in diabetics is 1.2 %. These studies were mainly surgical, in that the patients were potential candidates for vitrectomy. It is possible that the incidence of VMT in a nonsurgical setting is lower, as patients with VMT may be more likely to consider vitrectomy than those without. Conversely, there may be a large number of cases where VMA coexists with DME, and this adhesion has some biological interplay with DME, even if the magnitude of that effect is difficult to quantify.

Conclusion

Vitreo-macular adhesion or VMT coexist with a number of retinal disorders at differing proportions. Figure 2.1 is a schematic representation of the different disorders that contribute to the overall burden of symptomatic VMA, and Table 2.2 summarizes the data. As can be seen from Table 2.2, the prevalence of retinal disease occurring in association with VMA is 1,574.2 per 100,000, with an annual incidence of 31.3 per 100,000. This prevalence figure is driven largely by the high prevalence of ERM detected in population-based studies, but it is not known how many of these cases were symptomatic. A more conservative approach would be to exclude the ERM prevalence figure, which results in a prevalence of 355.2 per 100,000.

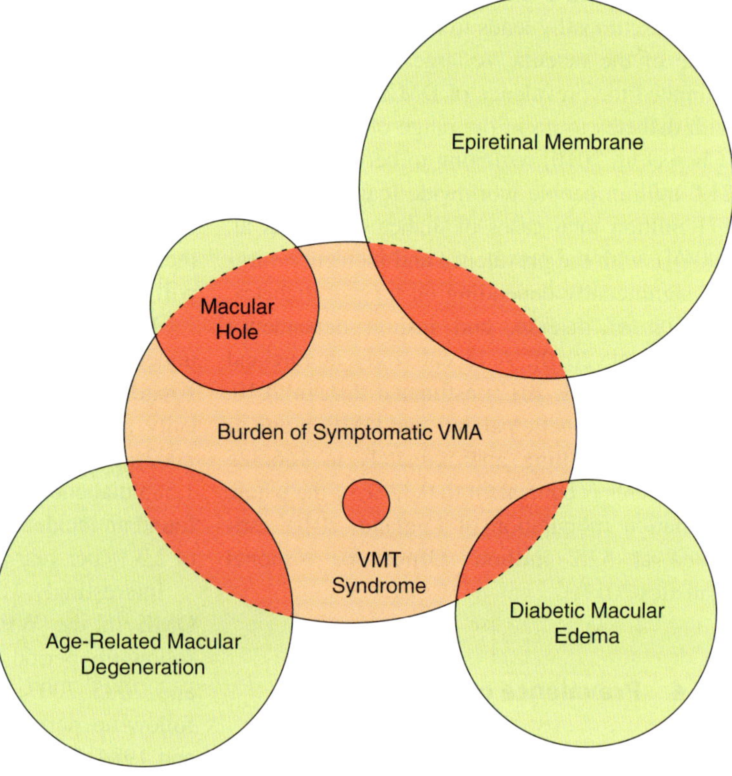

Fig. 2.1 Schematic diagram representing the association of vitreo-macular adhesion (VMA) and vitreo-macular traction (VMT) with several retinal conditions. The areas shaded in *red* represent those diseases in which VMA or VMT either cause or is associated with retinal disease. The area of each circle reflects the prevalence of the disease, and the area of overlap with symptomatic VMA is based on the proportion of that disease known to have either VMA or VMT. The figure is based on the data presented in Tables 2.1 and 2.2. The prevalence of epiretinal membrane is underrepresented in the figure, as many cases of epiretinal membrane detected in population studies may have been asymptomatic.

Table 2.2 Summary of Estimated Prevalence and Incidence of VMA

Condition	Proportion associated with VMA (%)	Prevalence of disease occurring in association with VMA (per 100,000 population)	Annual incidence of disease occurring in association with VMA (per 100,000 population)
Macular hole	72.8 (Hikichi et al. 1995)	108	6.4
Epiretinal membrane	12.7 (Appiah et al. 1988; Hirokawa et al. 1986)	1,219	0.4
VMT syndrome	100 (by definition of disease)	22.5	0.56
Wet AMD	16.7 (Jackson et al. 2012)	170.3	23.9
DME	17 (Jackson et al. 2012)	54.4	–
Total[a]	–	1,574.2	31.3

[a]These calculations were performed using the weighted averages for each condition shown in Table 2.1, multiplied by the current evidence available regarding the proportion of cases that occur in association with vitreo-macular adhesion (VMA)

This may better reflect the true prevalence of symptomatic VMA. Note that this figure excludes diseases for which the incidence or prevalence is not known. Including these cases would increase the burden of symptomatic VMA.

It is important to understand the limitations of our attempt to generate an overall figure summarizing the burden of disease associated with symptomatic VMA. In several cases we made an estimate based on inferred or incomplete data, as that was all that was possible. Another important limitation relates to causation. In the case of VMT syndrome the disease can be wholly attributed to symptomatic VMA. For wet AMD there is strong evidence of an association, but that does not mean that VMA aggravates or causes wet AMD, even if that remains a possibility. For DME even the association is uncertain. In the case of ERM it seems likely that ERM and VMT often coexist, but relief of VMT may not in itself be enough to relieve symptoms, if residual membranes lead to persisting macular distortion. Therefore, this chapter should be seen as a very broad overview of the *association* between VMA and various important retinal diseases rather than an attempt to summarize the burden of disease *attributable* to VMA. There are many other caveats to this analysis, as outlined in each section of the chapter. These caveats mean that the final figure must be taken as a very approximate estimate as, at present, the data do not allow for a more accurate assessment.

As our understanding of VMA and VMT increases, especially their relationship with AMD and DME, the true magnitude of the burden of disease will hopefully become more apparent. With the established technique of vitrectomy, and the promising new approach of pharmacologic vitreolysis, interest in VMA is likely to increase, and hopefully with that new treatment options will emerge to decrease the global burden of symptomatic VMA.

Compliance with Ethical Requirements Dr Jackson is a consultant for Alcon, Bausch & Lomb, Mesoblast, and Thrombogenics and has received research grant support from NeoVista, Novartis, and Oraya. Dr Simpson has no conflicts of interest. No animal or human studies were carried out by the authors for this chapter.

References

Appiah AP, Hirose T, Kado M (1988) A review of 324 cases of idiopathic premacular gliosis. Am J Ophthalmol 106(5):533–535

Bunce C, Wormald R (2008) Causes of blind certifications in England and Wales: April 1999-March 2000. Eye (Lond) 22(7):905–911

Chauhan DS, Antcliff RJ, Rai PA, Williamson TH, Marshall J (2000) Papillofoveal traction in macular hole formation: the role of optical coherence tomography. Arch Ophthalmol 118(1):32–38

Chen E, Looman M, Laouri M, Gallagher M, Van Nuys K, Lakdawalla D, Fortuny J (2010) Burden of illness of diabetic macular edema: literature review. Curr Med Res Opin 26(7):1587–1597

Davis MD, Blodi BA (2001) Proliferative diabetic retinopathy. In: Schachat AP (ed) Retina, vol 2. Mosby, St Louis, pp 1315–1316

European Population Statistics (2012) European Commission – eurostat. http://epp.eurostat.ec.europa.eu/portal/page/portal/population/data/main_tables. Accessed 1 May 2012

Foos RY (1977) Vitreoretinal juncture; epiretinal membranes and vitreous. Invest Ophthalmol Vis Sci 16(5):416–422

Friedman DS, O'Colmain BJ, Munoz B, Tomany SC, McCarty C, de Jong PT, Nemesure B, Mitchell P, Kempen J (2004) Prevalence of age-related macular degeneration in the United States. Arch Ophthalmol 122(4):564–572

Gallemore RP, Jumper JM, McCuen BW 2nd, Jaffe GJ, Postel EA, Toth CA (2000) Diagnosis of vitreoretinal adhesions in macular disease with optical coherence tomography. Retina 20(2):115–120

Gass JD (1988) Idiopathic senile macular hole. Its early stages and pathogenesis. Arch Ophthalmol 106(5):629–639

Gass JD (1995) Reappraisal of biomicroscopic classification of stages of development of a macular hole. Am J Ophthalmol 119(6):752–759

Gaudric A, Haouchine B, Massin P, Paques M, Blain P, Erginay A (1999) Macular hole formation: new data provided by optical coherence tomography. Arch Ophthalmol 117(6):744–751

Harbour JW, Smiddy WE, Flynn HW Jr, Rubsamen PE (1996) Vitrectomy for diabetic macular edema associated with a thickened and taut posterior hyaloid membrane. Am J Ophthalmol 121(4):405–413

Hee MR, Puliafito CA, Wong C, Duker JS, Reichel E, Schuman JS, Swanson EA, Fujimoto JG (1995) Optical coherence tomography of macular holes. Ophthalmology 102(5):748–756

Henricsson M, Sellman A, Tyrberg M, Groop L (1999) Progression to proliferative retinopathy and macular oedema requiring treatment. Assessment of the alternative classification of the Wisconsin Study. Acta Ophthalmol Scand 77(2):218–223

Hikichi T, Yoshida A, Akiba J, Trempe CL (1995) Natural outcomes of stage 1, 2, 3, and 4 idiopathic macular holes. Br J Ophthalmol 79(6):517–520

Hirokawa H, Jalkh AE, Takahashi M, Takahashi M, Trempe CL, Schepens CL (1986) Role of the vitreous in idiopathic preretinal macular fibrosis. Am J Ophthalmol 101(2):166–169

Hospital Episode Statistics (2012) Main procedures and interventions. http://www.hesonline.nhs.uk. Accessed 1 May 2012

Jackson TL, Donachie PH, Sparrow JM, Johnston RL (2013) United Kingdom National Ophthalmology Database Study of Vitreoretinal Surgery: Report 1; Case mix, complications, and cataract. Eye 27: 644-651

Jackson TL, Nicod E, Angelis A, Grimaccia F, Prevost AT, Simpson AR, Kanavos P (2012) Vitreous attachment in age-related macular degeneration, diabetic macular edema, and retinal vein occlusion: a systematic review and meta-analysis. Retina 33(6):1099–1108

Johnson RN, Gass JD (1988) Idiopathic macular holes. Observations, stages of formation, and implications for surgical intervention. Ophthalmology 95(7):917–924

King H, Aubert RE, Herman WH (1998) Global burden of diabetes, 1995–2025: prevalence, numerical estimates, and projections. Diabetes Care 21(9): 1414–1431

Klaver CC, Wolfs RC, Vingerling JR, Hofman A, de Jong PT (1998) Age-specific prevalence and causes of blindness and visual impairment in an older population: the Rotterdam Study. Arch Ophthalmol 116(5):653–658

Klaver CC, Assink JJ, van Leeuwen R, Wolfs RC, Vingerling JR, Stijnen T, Hofman A, de Jong PT (2001) Incidence and progression rates of age-related maculopathy: the Rotterdam Study. Invest Ophthalmol Vis Sci 42(10):2237–2241

Klein R, Klein BE, Moss SE, Davis MD, DeMets DL (1984) The Wisconsin epidemiologic study of diabetic retinopathy. IV. Diabetic macular edema. Ophthalmology 91(12):1464–1474

Klein R, Klein BE, Linton KL, De Mets DL (1991) The Beaver Dam Eye Study: visual acuity. Ophthalmology 98(8):1310–1315

Klein R, Klein BE, Wang Q, Moss SE (1994) The epidemiology of epiretinal membranes. Trans Am Ophthalmol Soc 92:403–425, discussion 425–430

Klein R, Klein BE, Jensen SC, Meuer SM (1997) The five-year incidence and progression of age-related maculopathy: the Beaver Dam Eye Study. Ophthalmology 104(1):7–21

Klein R, Klein BE, Tomany SC, Meuer SM, Huang GH (2002) Ten-year incidence and progression of age-related maculopathy: The Beaver Dam eye study. Ophthalmology 109(10):1767–1779

Klein R, Knudtson MD, Lee KE, Gangnon R, Klein BE (2009) The Wisconsin Epidemiologic Study of Diabetic Retinopathy XXIII: the twenty-five-year incidence of macular edema in persons with type 1 diabetes. Ophthalmology 116(3):497–503

la Cour M, Friis J (2002) Macular holes: classification, epidemiology, natural history and treatment. Acta Ophthalmol Scand 80(6):579–587

Laidlaw DA (2008) Vitrectomy for diabetic macular oedema. Eye (Lond) 22(10):1337–1341

Lewis H, Abrams GW, Blumenkranz MS, Campo RV (1992) Vitrectomy for diabetic macular traction and edema associated with posterior hyaloidal traction. Ophthalmology 99(5):753–759

Ling R, Ramsewak V, Taylor D, Jacob J (2002) Longitudinal study of a cohort of people with diabetes screened by the Exeter Diabetic Retinopathy Screening Programme. Eye (Lond) 16(2):140–145

Lister W (1924) Holes in the retina and their clinical significance. Br J Ophthalmol 8(1):i4–i20

Margherio RR, Trese MT, Margherio AR, Cartright K (1989) Surgical management of vitreomacular traction syndromes. Ophthalmology 96(9):1437–1445

McCannel CA, Ensminger JL, Diehl NN, Hodge DN (2009) Population-based incidence of macular holes. Ophthalmology 116(7):1366–1369

McDonald HR, Johnson RN, Schatz H (1994) Surgical results in the vitreomacular traction syndrome. Ophthalmology 101(8):1397–1402, discussion 1403

Melberg NS, Williams DF, Balles MW, Jaffe GJ, Meredith TA, Sneed SR, Westrich DJ (1995) Vitrectomy for vitreomacular traction syndrome with macular detachment. Retina 15(3):192–197

Minassian DC, Owens DR, Reidy A (2012) Prevalence of diabetic macular oedema and related health and social care resource use in England. Br J Ophthalmol 96(3):345–349

Mitchell P, Smith W, Chey T, Wang JJ, Chang A (1997) Prevalence and associations of epiretinal membranes. The Blue Mountains Eye Study, Australia. Ophthalmology 104(6):1033–1040

Mitchell P, Wang JJ, Foran S, Smith W (2002) Five-year incidence of age-related maculopathy lesions: the Blue Mountains Eye Study. Ophthalmology 109(6): 1092–1097

Miyazaki M, Kiyohara Y, Yoshida A, Iida M, Nose Y, Ishibashi T (2005) The 5-year incidence and risk factors for age-related maculopathy in a general Japanese population: the Hisayama study. Invest Ophthalmol Vis Sci 46(6):1907–1910

Munoz B, West SK, Rubin GS, Schein OD, Quigley HA, Bressler SB, Bandeen-Roche K (2000) Causes of blindness and visual impairment in a population of older Americans: The Salisbury Eye Evaluation Study. Arch Ophthalmol 118(6):819–825

Nasrallah FP, Jalkh AE, Van Coppenolle F, Kado M, Trempe CL, McMeel JW, Schepens CL (1988) The role of the vitreous in diabetic macular edema. Ophthalmology 95(10):1335–1339

Office for National Statistics (2011) Population estimates for UK, England and Wales, Scotland and Northern Ireland – Mid-2010. http://www.ons.gov.uk/ons/taxonomy/index.html?nscl=Population. Accessed 1 May 2012

Owen CG, Jarrar Z, Wormald R, Cook DG, Fletcher AE, Rudnicka AR (2012) The estimated prevalence and incidence of late stage age related macular degeneration in the UK. Br J Ophthalmol 96(5):752–756

Pendergast SD (1998) Vitrectomy for diabetic macular edema associated with a taut premacular posterior hyaloid. Curr Opin Ophthalmol 9(3):71–75

Pendergast SD, Hassan TS, Williams GA, Cox MS, Margherio RR, Ferrone PJ, Garretson BR, Trese MT (2000) Vitrectomy for diffuse diabetic macular edema associated with a taut premacular posterior hyaloid. Am J Ophthalmol 130(2):178–186

Rahmani B, Tielsch JM, Katz J, Gottsch J, Quigley H, Javitt J, Sommer A (1996) The cause-specific prevalence of visual impairment in an urban population. The Baltimore Eye Survey. Ophthalmology 103(11): 1721–1726

Reese AB, Jones IS, Cooper WC (1967) Macular changes secondary to vitreous traction. Am J Ophthalmol 64(3):544–549

Reese AB, Jones IS, Cooper WC (1970) Vitreomacular traction syndrome confirmed histologically. Am J Ophthalmol 69(6):975–977

Rossing P (2005) The changing epidemiology of diabetic microangiopathy in type 1 diabetes. Diabetologia 48(8):1439–1444

Sen P, Bhargava A, Vijaya L, George R (2008) Prevalence of idiopathic macular hole in adult rural and urban south Indian population. Clin Experiment Ophthalmol 36(3):257–260

Sidd RJ, Fine SL, Owens SL, Patz A (1982) Idiopathic preretinal gliosis. Am J Ophthalmol 94(1):44–48

Simpson ARH, Petraca R, Jackson TL (2012) Vitreomacular adhesion and neovascular age-related macular degeneration. Surv Ophthalmol 57(6): 498–509

Smiddy WE, Michels RG, Glaser BM, deBustros S (1988) Vitrectomy for macular traction caused by incomplete vitreous separation. Arch Ophthalmol 106(5): 624–628

Sommer A, Tielsch JM, Katz J, Quigley HA, Gottsch JD, Javitt JC, Martone JF, Royall RM, Witt KA, Ezrine S (1991) Racial differences in the cause-specific prevalence of blindness in east Baltimore. N Engl J Med 325(20):1412–1417

Tanner V, Chauhan DS, Jackson TL, Williamson TH (2001) Optical coherence tomography of the vitreoretinal interface in macular hole formation. Br J Ophthalmol 85(9):1092–1097

The 2012 Statistical Abstract (2012) United States Census Bureau. http://www.census.gov/compendia/statab/cats/population.html. Accessed 1 May 2012

van Effenterre G, Guyot-Argenton C, Guiberteau B, Hany I, Lacotte JL (1993) Macular edema caused by contraction of the posterior hyaloid in diabetic retinopathy. Surgical treatment of a series of 22 cases. J Fr Ophtalmol 16(11):602–610

Wang JJ, Foran S, Mitchell P (2000) Age-specific prevalence and causes of bilateral and unilateral visual impairment in older Australians: the Blue Mountains Eye Study. Clin Experiment Ophthalmol 28(4):268–273

Wang S, Xu L, Jonas JB (2006) Prevalence of full-thickness macular holes in urban and rural adult Chinese: the Beijing Eye Study. Am J Ophthalmol 141(3):589–591

Wang JJ, Rochtchina E, Lee AJ, Chia EM, Smith W, Cumming RG, Mitchell P (2007) Ten-year incidence and progression of age-related maculopathy: the blue Mountains Eye Study. Ophthalmology 114(1): 92–98

Weih LM, VanNewkirk MR, McCarty CA, Taylor HR (2000) Age-specific causes of bilateral visual impairment. Arch Ophthalmol 118(2):264–269

Wild S, Roglic G, Green A, Sicree R, King H (2004) Global prevalence of diabetes: estimates for the year 2000 and projections for 2030. Diabetes Care 27(5):1047–1053

Wise GN (1975) Relationship of idiopathic preretinal macular fibrosis to posterior vitreous detachment. Am J Ophthalmol 79(3):358–362

Wiznia RA (1986) Posterior vitreous detachment and idiopathic preretinal macular gliosis. Am J Ophthalmol 102(2):196–198

Anatomy and Physiology of the Vitreo-macular Interface

3

Amitha Domalpally, Sapna Gangaputra, and Ronald P. Danis

3.1 History

The vitreous humor (*vitreus*, glassy; *humor*, fluid) has been recognized as a distinct anatomic structure since the ancient times (Duke-Elder and Wybar 1961). The first attempts to systematically describe the vitreous anatomy were seen in mid-eighteenth-century observations (Duke-Elder and Wybar 1961). Microscopic studies on the vitreous began in mid-nineteenth century leading to differing interpretations about the structure of the vitreous. Much of the controversy was related to the difficulties with microscopic preparation of the vitreous due to its high water content and difficulties with staining and fixation, which led to highly variable specimen appearances (Wolf 1968). The fibrillar structure of the vitreous seen on slit lamp biomicroscopy further added to speculation on vitreous structure. Theories by notable anatomists were advanced, such as the alveolar theory by Demours, the lamellar theory by Zinn, the radial theory by Hannover, and the fibrillar theory by Schwalbe (Sebag 1989d;

Duke-Elder and Wybar 1961). Early descriptions of the vitreous structure identified a "hyaloid membrane" within which the vitreous was enveloped. By the early twentieth century, the hyaloid membrane was shown to be a condensation of the vitreous rather than a true membrane, and the term "vitreous cortex" was coined.

3.2 Embryology

The primary vitreous begins to develop during the third to fourth week of gestation. In the optic cup, a space formed by the separation of neuroectoderm from the surface ectoderm is filled with PAS-positive fibrillar structures, arranged parallel to the developing retina. The hyaloid artery system grows into the primary vitreous through the optic stalk to reach the fibrous capsule surrounding the lens (Sebag 1989b; Tolentino et al. 1976).

The secondary vitreous forms between 6 weeks and 3 months of development and is the main contributor to the adult vitreous. The secondary vitreous develops entirely from neural ectoderm and collapses the primary vitreous forwards. The demarcation between the primary and secondary vitreous is visible until the third month of gestation and ultimately transforms into the walls of the Cloquet's canal. The concept of a distinct primary and secondary vitreous has been questioned in recent times, giving rise to the theory that primary vitreous remodels into the secondary vitreous (Ponsioen et al. 2010). Around the third month, the vitreous base is

A. Domalpally, MD • S. Gangaputra, MD, MPH
Department of Ophthalmology and Visual Sciences, University of Wisconsin-Madison, Madison, WI, USA

R.P. Danis, MD (✉)
Department of Ophthalmology and Visual Sciences, University of Wisconsin-Madison, Madison, WI, USA

University of Wisconsin Fundus Photograph Reading Center, University of Wisconsin-Madison, 8010 Excelsior Drive, Suite 100, Madison, WI 53717, USA
e-mail: rdanis@rc.ophth.wisc.edu

A. Girach, M.D. de Smet (eds.), *Diseases of the Vitreo-Macular Interface*, Essentials in Ophthalmology, DOI 10.1007/978-3-642-40034-6_3, © Springer-Verlag Berlin Heidelberg 2014

visible as a condensed annular ring. The hyaloid artery gradually atrophies but remains as a thin-walled structure within the vitreous, detaching from the optic disc by the eighth month (Tolentino et al. 1976).

A tertiary vitreous has been described but is generally considered a misnomer because it is derived from the developing ciliary body and is a part of the zonular system.

3.3 Anatomy

With a volume of approximately 4.0 ml, the vitreous occupies about four fifths the volume of the eye. The axial length of the vitreous is about 16 mm in an adult emmetropic eye (Sebag 1989d; Larsen 1971). It is spherical posteriorly and has a depression anteriorly corresponding to the lens, called the patellar fossa. The vitreous body consists of the vitreous base, the vitreous cortex, and the core vitreous (Fig. 3.1).

The vitreous base is a three-dimensional structure, dense in collagen, extending 1.5–2 mm anterior to ora serrata and 1–3 mm posterior to the ora serrata (Hogan 1963). The border extends more posteriorly temporally than nasally. The vitreous cortex (or the hyaloid membrane) envelopes the vitreous body and is 100–200 μm in thickness (Tolentino et al. 1976). It is divided into anterior and posterior parts by the vitreous base. The cortex is thin over the macula and absent over the optic nerve (Sebag 1992). The vitreous cortex is attached to all its contiguous structures with the strongest connection at the vitreous base. At the vitreous base, the vitreous fibers change their parallel orientation to the retina and splay out to attach perpendicularly to the anterior and posterior borders of the vitreous base (Green and Sebag 2001).

Other prominent vitreoretinal attachments include the lens, the retinal parafoveal area, and the margin of the optic nerve head and along major retinal blood vessels (Fig. 3.2). The

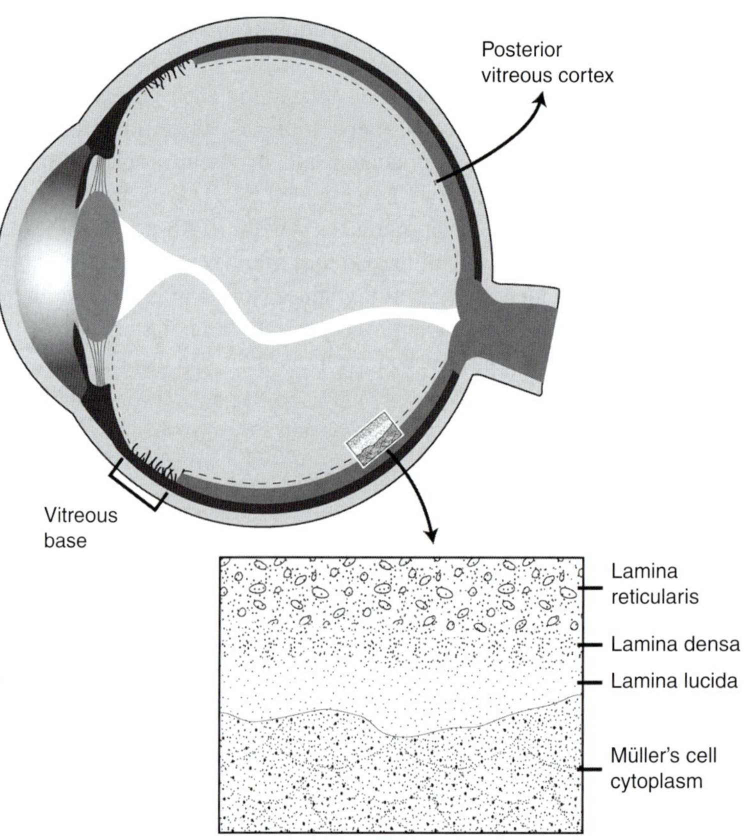

Fig. 3.1 Schematic diagram showing the layers of the vitreoretinal interface

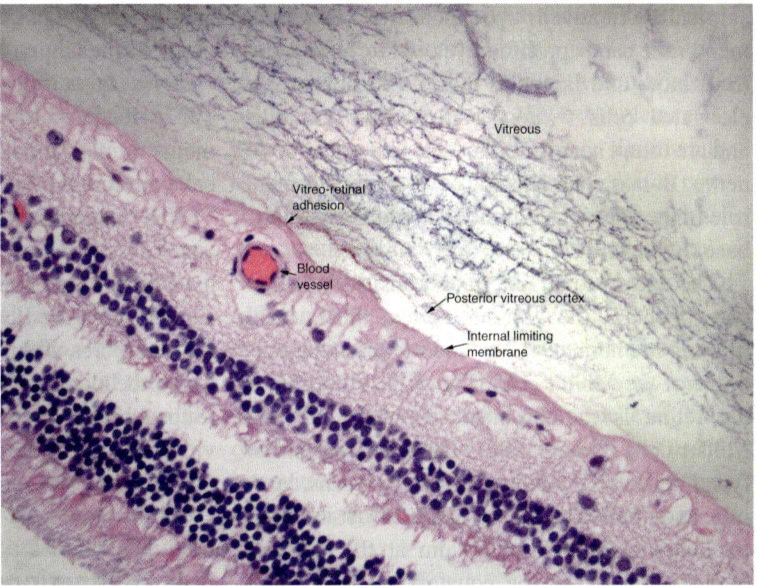

Fig. 3.2 Histological section of the posterior cortex showing fine eosinophilic vitreous fibrils attached to a blood vessel (H&E 20X) (courtesy of Potter H)

attachments and spaces with them have been named after the anatomists or histologists who discovered them. The Wieger's ligament of the lens is a circular area of attachment between the vitreous cortex and the posterior lens capsule. The space enclosed within Wieger's ligament is known as the space of Berger. It has been proposed that this space is in continuation with Cloquet's canal and opens into the space of Martegiani around the optic nerve. Recent studies have disputed the evidence for these channels within the vitreous (Los et al. 2000). In an eye with complete posterior vitreous detachment, a floating intact or disrupted ring corresponding to the optic nerve can often be visualized. Remnants of the peripapillary glial tissue attached to the posterior vitreous cortex around the optic nerve form the Weiss' ring.

The vitreous cortex is composed of three main elements – collagen fibers, fibrocytic and macrophagic cells, and complex mucopolysaccharides (Tolentino et al. 1976; Hogan 1963). Ultrastructurally, the core vitreous resembles the vitreous cortex but contains less dense structures (Fig. 3.2) (Sebag 1992) . The fibers in the vitreous cortex are collagenous and oriented in an anteroposterior direction. The fibers insert at the vitreous base anteriorly, and the posterior insertions are at the posterior cortex in the region of the macula (Sebag 1989d; Green 1985). Parallel bundles of collagen traverse without branching but network with each other; an individual collagen fibril may deviate from one bundle to join an adjacent bundle (Sebag 1992; Bishop et al. 2004). The space between the bundles is filled with mucopolysaccharides consisting mainly of large hyaluronic acid molecules (Tolentino et al. 1976; Sebag and Balazs 1989). The organized collagen fibrils with intervening hyaluronic acid are responsible for the gel state of the vitreous (Bishop et al. 2004).

Hyalocytes account for 90 % of vitreous cells and fibroblasts for the remaining 10 % (Ponsioen et al. 2010). Hyalocytes have a lobulated nucleus, a moderate amount of mitochondria, and PAS-positive granules. Their shape varies from round or oval to an irregular shape with cytoplasmic projections. Amoeboid movements of the whole cell within the vitreous have been demonstrated (Balazs et al. 1964). The cells are concentrated at the peripheral vitreous, at the vitreous base, along the posterior pole and blood vessels and appear to be important in maintaining the vitreous clear and avascular through vitreous cavity immune modulation (Ponsioen et al. 2010; Noda et al. 2004; Sakamoto and Ishibashi 2011). Hyalocytes have also been implicated in exacerbation of ocular inflammation and found in

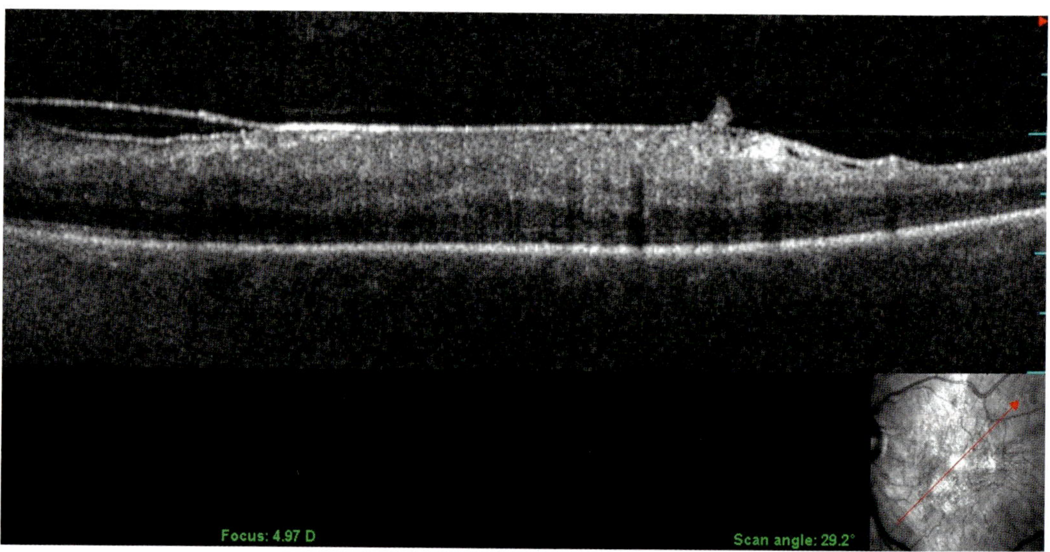

Fig. 4.11 Vitreoschisis. Combined OCT-SLO imaging demonstrates a split in the posterior vitreous cortex as a result of anomalous PVD. Histopathology of this specimen confirmed the presence of vitreoschisis (Reprinted from Gupta et al (2011)

4.4.2.1 Peripheral Anomalous PVD: Retinal Tears and Detachment

Autopsy studies found that PVD is associated with retinal breaks in 14.3 % of all cases. Lindner (Lindner 1937) found minimal vitreous hemorrhage in 13–19 % of cases with PVD. Nondiabetic patients with fundus-obscuring vitreous hemorrhage have a high-incidence of retinal tears (67 %) and retinal detachments (39 %) (Sarrafizadeh et al. 2001).

4.4.2.2 Posterior Anomalous PVD and Vitreo-macular Adhesion (VMA)

The clinical manifestations of VMA and surgical management of the vitreo-macular traction syndrome (VMTS) have been previously described (Smiddy et al. 1988; Sebag et al. 1994), VMA is also important in patients with age-related macular degeneration (AMD), the leading cause of blindness in elderly individuals. Recent studies (Krebs et al. 2007; Robison et al. 2009), have identified that true PVD is protective against wet AMD, while anomalous PVD with persistent VMA promotes choroidal neovascularization. VMA is also important in diabetic macular edema, the leading cause of blindness in young and middle-aged individuals.

4.4.2.3 Vitreoschisis

Kishi and colleagues (Kishi et al. 1986) reported that PVD was associated with vitreous cortex remnants at the fovea in 26 of 59 (44 %) human eyes studied at autopsy with scanning electron microscopy. When these remnants are a layer or sheet of posterior vitreous cortex, the term *vitreoschisis* is appropriate. On clinical examination, the inner wall of the vitreoschisis cavity may be clinically confused with a PVD when the posterior layer of the split vitreous cortex remains attached to the ILL of the retina. Ultrasonography can at times detect the split layers in vitreoschisis, depending upon the thickness of the layers. Studies (Chu et al. 1996) detected vitreoschisis by ultrasound in 20 % of eyes with proliferative diabetic retinopathy. Recent studies (Gupta et al. 2011) employing OCT/SLO detected vitreoschisis in about half of patients with macular pucker and macular holes (Fig. 4.11).

Vitreo-macular Adhesion (VMA) and Macular Pucker

Following vitreoschisis, premacular membranes can contract causing visual impairment and metamorphopsia. Studies of excised tissue have demonstrated the presence of astrocytes and RPE cells (Michels 1982; Smiddy et al. 1989), but

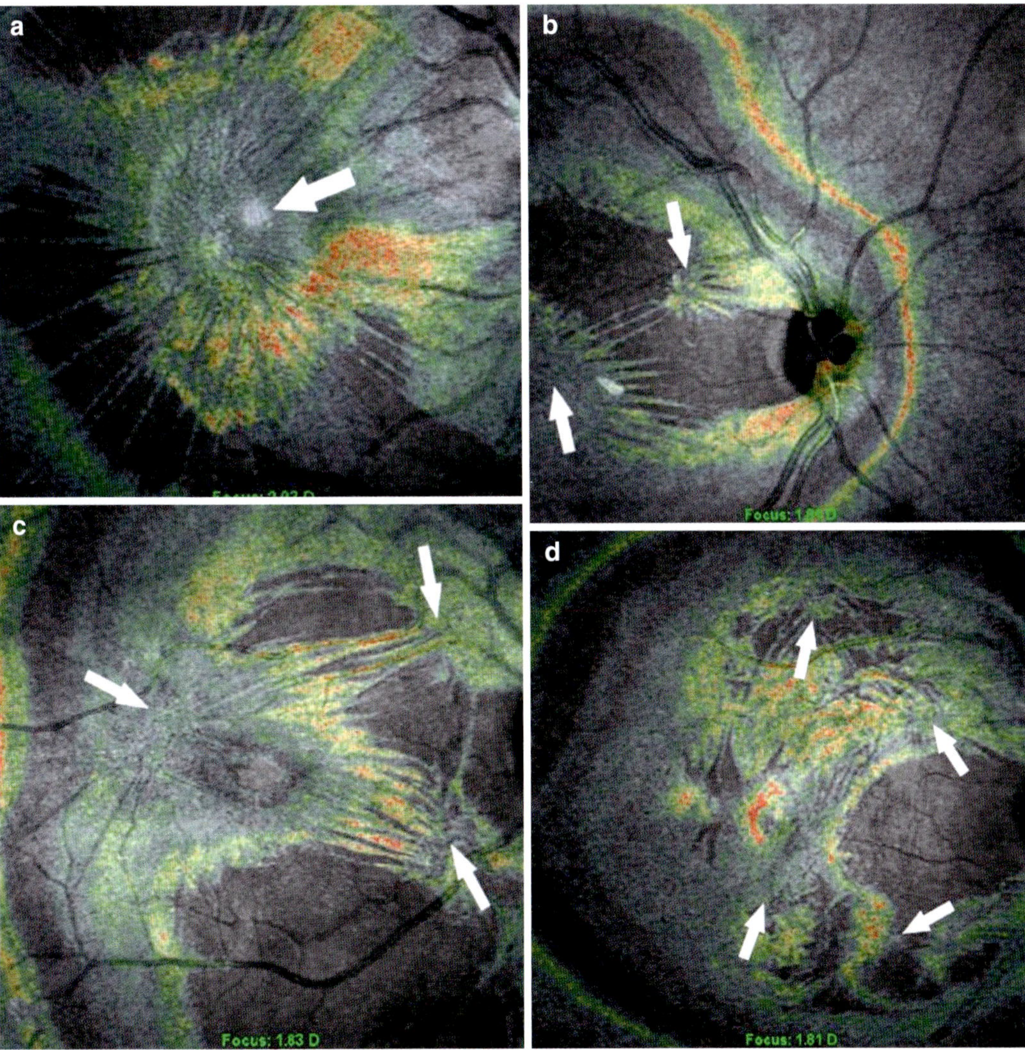

Fig. 4.12 Multifocal retinal contraction in macular pucker. Superimposed coronal plane OCT images upon the SLO fundus images reveal multi-focality (*arrows*) in the pattern of macular pucker. (**a**) 1 pucker center; (**b**) 2 pucker centers; (**c**): 3 pucker centers; (**d**) 4 puckers centers. See Gupta et al. 2008

there are likely to be hyalocytes as well. It has been hypothesized that macular pucker results when vitreoschisis splits the cortex anterior to hyalocytes leaving a cellular membrane attached to the macula (Gupta et al. 2011). The hyalocytes then elicit migration of monocytes from the circulation and contraction of vitreous via the action of CTGF (Hiryama et al. 2004). Recent studies (Gupta et al. 2008) have also identified that nearly half of all eyes with macular pucker have more than one site of retinal contraction (Fig. 4.12). There is a higher incidence of intraretinal cysts and significantly more macular thickening with increasing foci of retinal contraction.

Vitreo-macular Adhesion and Macular Holes

The precise pathogenesis of macular holes is unknown, although there are several hypotheses (Schumann et al. 2006; Sebag et al. 1994), such as anteroposterior traction by vitreous fibers and tangential traction upon the macula. While the ILL of the retina could induce such traction, noninvasive imaging studies with combined

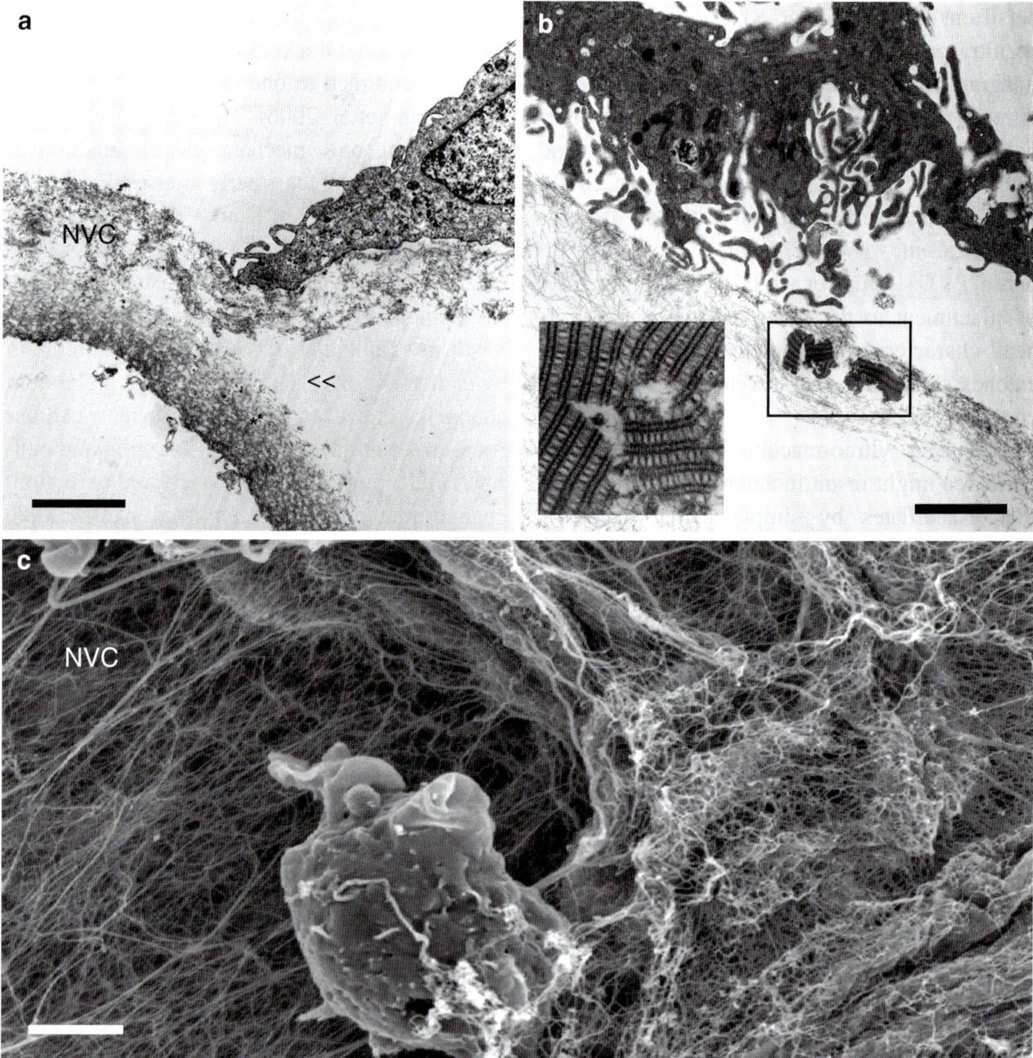

Fig. 5.2 Vitreoschisis with residual vitreous cortex collagen. Transmission electron micrographs of (**a**) an ultrathin section presenting a thick layer of vitreous cortex collagen, also called native vitreous collagen (NVC), that is partially directly situated on the internal limiting membrane (ILM) (*asterisk*) and partially detached (*arrows*) from the ILM, and (**b**) an ultrathin section demonstrating compact fibrous long-spacing collagen (FLSC) (*rectangle*) within a vitreous collagen layer as morphological evidence for vitreous collagen degradation and remodelling. Insert shows FLSC characterised by transverse banding and typical periodicity at higher magnification. (**c**) Scanning electron micrograph presents the vitreal side of the ILM with masses of vitreous collagen fibrils (NVC) after vitreoschisis (Specimens were surgically removed during vitrectomy from eyes with macular pucker at the Department of Ophthalmology, Ludwig-Maximilians-University Munich, Germany. Original magnification: (a) and (b) ×4,800, scale bar = 2.1 μm; insert ×28,500; (c) ×4,000, scale bar = 2.5 μm)

Sebag et al. 2007; Schwartz et al. 1996). Electron microscopic studies with ultrastructural evaluation of surgically excised ILM specimens were particularly precise in the demonstration of vitreous collagen fibrils on the ILM. Even small amounts of single collagen fibres can be detected by transmission or scanning electron microscopy. Ultrastructural evidence for vitreoschisis was repeatedly reported, e.g. in eyes with macular holes, macular pucker, vitreo-macular traction syndrome, and diabetic macular oedema (Gandorfer et al. 2002; Schumann et al. 2006, 2008; Gandorfer 2007). In eyes with vitreoschisis, fibrocellular proliferation is mostly directly situated on a continuous layer of vitreous cortex collagen or embedded in cortical vitreous collagen remnants on the ILM (Schumann et al. 2006; Green 2006).

5.3.1 Degradation of Vitreous Cortex Collagen

Structure and composition of vitreous collagen fibrils underlie age-related changes that influence the content of growth factors, cytokines, and enzymes as well as the ability of cells to interact with vitreous collagen (Bishop et al. 2004). In this context, enzymatic vitreous collagen degradation was suggested to participate in mechanisms of age-related liquefaction. Studies on the activity of vitreous matrix metalloproteinases and the presence of abnormal collagen variants within vitreous collagen support the hypothesis of collagen degradation.

Abnormal collagen variants such as fibrous and segment compact long-spacing collagen within remnants of cortical vitreous were reported by ultrastructural evaluation of surgically excised ILM specimens from various traction vitreo-maculopathies. Compact long-spacing collagen is a fibrillar precipitate of collagen molecules that are noticeably thicker than normal collagen fibrils and are characterised by transverse banding. It was found in pathologic tissue and represents an intermediate stage of collagen in the degradation of normal collagen fibrils (Dingemans and Teeling 1994; Ishida et al. 2000; Eyden and Tzaphlidou 2001). The presence of long-spacing collagen demonstrates morphological evidence of a remodelling process of premacular vitreous cortex that was reported in idiopathic macular holes, lamellar macular holes, macular pucker, vitreo-macular traction syndrome, and myopic foveoschisis (Messmer et al. 1998; Shinoda et al. 2000; Schumann et al. 2006; Parolini et al. 2011; Bando et al. 2005). Vitreous collagen degradation may potentially result from alterations of

cell-cell and cell-matrix interactions in the context of age-related vitreous changes which may facilitate splitting of the posterior vitreous cortex layers.

5.3.2 Vitreous Cortex Remnants on the Internal Limiting Membrane

Dependent upon the level of split in vitreoschisis, there are differences in the thickness of cortical vitreous layers that are left behind at the macula. Sebag hypothesised that a thick, cellular membrane remains attached to the ILM if the split occurs anterior to the level of hyalocytes, whereas a thin, acellular membrane remains attached to the ILM if the split occurs posterior to the hyalocytes (Sebag 2008). In the first condition, inward (centripetal) contraction of the membrane induces macular pucker, whereas the second condition with outward (centrifugal) tangential contraction induces macular holes and cystoid spaces in vitreo-maculopathies.

However, epiretinal membrane contraction is not a collagen-based process. Traction is generated by cellular components that possess contractile properties at the vitreoretinal interface (Kampik et al. 1980). Most importantly, the presence of vitreous cortex remnants on the ILM in vitreoschisis supports cell migration. Consequently, epiretinal cell proliferation on vitreous cortex remnants may result in fibrocellular or fibrovascular epiretinal membrane formation causing vitreo-macular traction. This phenomenon has not only been shown in macular holes, macular pucker, and vitreo-macular traction syndrome but also in diabetic eyes that are clinically often characterised by a thickened and taut cortical vitreous cortex (Sebag 1996; Gandorfer 2007).

Complete removal of vitreous cortex collagen from the retinal surface is critical for surgical success (Schumann et al. 2007, 2008). However, ultrastructural studies proved that mechanical separation of the vitreous cortex from the ILM remains incomplete. Vitreous cortex collagen left behind on the ILM after vitrectomy might serve as a scaffold for epiretinal cell migration and (re) proliferation causing formation of epiretinal membranes with vitreoretinal traction and surgical failure (Yoshida and Kishi 2007; Fekrat et al. 1995; Gandorfer 2009; Gandorfer et al. 2011).

5.4 Epiretinal Cell Proliferation

Proliferation of epiretinal cells on the ILM with epiretinal membrane formation is heterogeneous in aetiology. In case of vitreo-macular traction, epiretinal cell proliferation can cause retinal traction and vice versa, vitreo-macular traction itself might cause epiretinal cell proliferation. However, it is still unknown if epiretinal membranes are a secondary event or rather part of the primary pathophysiology of vitreo-macular disorders.

Furthermore, epiretinal cell proliferation with membrane formation is also heterogeneous in composition depending on the underlying stimulus. Morphological and immunocytochemical analyses of surgically excised ILM specimens have demonstrated a variety of cell phenotypes in epiretinal membranes including glial cells (retinal Müller cells, fibrous astrocytes, and microglia), hyalocytes, retinal pigment epithelial cells, fibrocytes, myofibroblasts, and blood-borne immune cells like macrophages (Kampik et al. 1980, 1981; Smiddy et al. 1989; Gandorfer et al. 2005; Schumann et al. 2006, 2011; Messmer et al. 1998; Gandorfer 2009; Hiscott et al. 1984a, 1984b). Moreover, neurite processes were demonstrated in epiretinal membranes of various etiologies suggesting neuronal remodelling capacity of the retina (Lesnik Oberstein et al. 2011). However, the definitive identification of epiretinal cells often appears difficult since phenotypic transdifferentiation with adoption of morphological features of other cell types and modified antigen expression complicates the determination of the cells' origin.

Two major hypotheses exist concerning the origin of proliferating epiretinal cells. Firstly, traction forces at the retina exerted by incomplete PVD allow for activation and migration of glial cells from the innermost retina to the surface of the ILM, where they are thought to proliferate and form epiretinal membranes (Bringmann and Wiedemann 2009). Secondly, age-related changes in the vitreous with vitreous gel liquefaction cause modifications of cell and collagen structures within the vitreous gel and cortex followed by migration and proliferation of hyalocytes on the vitreoretinal interface.

5.4.1 The Role of Retinal Glia

Anteroposterior and tangential traction forces can be transmitted from the vitreous to retinal Müller cells and astrocytes due to the close anatomic relationship between the internal limiting membrane and Müller cell footplates. Traction forces mediated by the ILM were shown to result in Müller glial cell activation (Kodal et al. 2000). Activated retinal Müller cells are considered to dedifferentiate, proliferate, and migrate from the retinal onto the vitreal side of the ILM. Dependent on pathogenic stimuli they further proliferate on the ILM and drive epiretinal membrane formation (Bringmann et al. 2006; Bringmann and Wiedemann 2009; Fisher and Lewis 2003). According to this theory, activated glial cells are believed to gain access to the retinal surface through pores or breaks in the ILM caused by PVD.

In fact, epiretinal membranes removed from traction maculopathies were demonstrated to contain glial fibrillary acidic protein (GFAP)-positive and vimentin-positive cells (Schumann et al. 2011; Vinores et al. 1990; Lewis and Fisher 2003). Both GFAP and vimentin are intermediate filament proteins that indicate glial cell activation in retinal injury (Nakazawa et al. 2007). By transmission electron microscopy, glial cell proliferation was shown to occur on the inner surface of cortical vitreous and even underneath the ILM in macular pucker (Gastaud et al. 2000; Heidenkummer and Kampik 1992; Haritoglou et al. 2007). Immunohistochemical investigations of retinal cell debris on the retinal side of the ILM demonstrated positive immunoreactivity for GFAP in correlation with the presence of epiretinal membranes (Kenawy et al. 2010). However, presence of glial cell proliferation underneath the ILM can be discussed in two ways. First, glial cells may proliferate in order to cross the ILM and promote epiretinal membrane formation, or second, gliosis underneath the ILM may be induced by epiretinal membranes themselves representing a secondary event.

There are findings that argue against the hypothesis that glial cells constitute the predominant cell type in epiretinal membranes. Histological studies reported that pores or breaks of the ILM are an extremely rare finding (Gandorfer et al. 2012). Only three pores of the ILM were found in 112 flat-mounted ILM specimens removed from eyes with idiopathic macular holes making it rather unlikely that a considerable number of glial cells migrate through the ILM to form epiretinal gliosis.

5.4.2 The Role of Hyalocytes

Hyalocytes are resident cells distributed in the vitreous cortex which are situated 20–50 μm anterior of the ILM (Hannover 1845; Balazs et al. 1964). Hyalocytes derive from the monocytes-macrophage lineage and represent resident macrophages that are usually in a quiescent stage as sentinel cells (Lazarus and Hageman 1994; Qiao et al. 2005). In the presence of pathologic stimuli, hyalocytes may undergo activation with still unknown specific or unspecific responses. The hyalocyte-specific antigens CD45 and CD64 were demonstrated in epiretinal cells of various traction maculopathies, including idiopathic macular holes, macular pucker, and vitreo-macular traction syndrome, pointing to the hypothesis that hyalocytes constitute a major cell type in the pathogenesis of vitreo-macular traction disorders.

Additionally, a significant number of epiretinal cells were found to present simultaneous positive immunoreactivity for GFAP and CD45 or CD64 (Schumann et al. 2011). Based on the co-localisation of glial cell and hyalocyte marker, it can be hypothesised that hyalocytes assume characteristics of glial cells or that glial cell debris and apoptotic glial cells were phagocytosed by activated hyalocytes. Thus, expression of the intermediate filament GFAP in epiretinal cells appears to be rather unspecific making GFAP-positive immunostaining alone no longer suitable to differentiate between glial or vitreal origin of cells.

Given that hyalocytes might adopt characteristics of glial cells thereby being more common in the composition of epiretinal membranes, we assume that transdifferentiated epiretinal cells in the vitreous cortex may be more frequent than previously thought and may have a greater variety of immunocytochemical properties than previously expected. This hypothesis suggests a substantial involvement of cell migration and cell proliferation in vitreo-macular traction disorders.

5.4.3 Cellular Elements of Contraction

Epiretinal membrane contraction is a cell mediated rather than a collagen-based process. Besides the hypothesis that contraction might be the consequence of migrating cells moving on a scaffold and applying traction through adhesion between cells and collagen (Grierson et al. 1996), there clearly is an important role of myofibroblasts in epiretinal membrane contraction. Myofibroblasts are a subset of fibroblasts distinguished by cytoplasmic aggregates of actin microfilaments forming stress bundles. Similar to smooth muscle cells, they are characterised by α-smooth muscle actin (α-SMA) immunoreactivity (Fig. 5.3). Cultured on collagen lattice, human myofibroblasts were shown to generate more potent traction forces than smooth muscle cells (Dallon and Ehrlich 2010). In vitreo-macular traction disorders such as macular pucker and vitreo-macular traction syndrome, myofibroblasts were reported to be predominating in cellular composition of epiretinal membranes (Gandorfer et al. 2002; Schumann et al. 2006).

Glial cells and hyalocytes were demonstrated to undergo myofibroblast-like transdifferentiation with positive α-SMA expression (Sakamoto

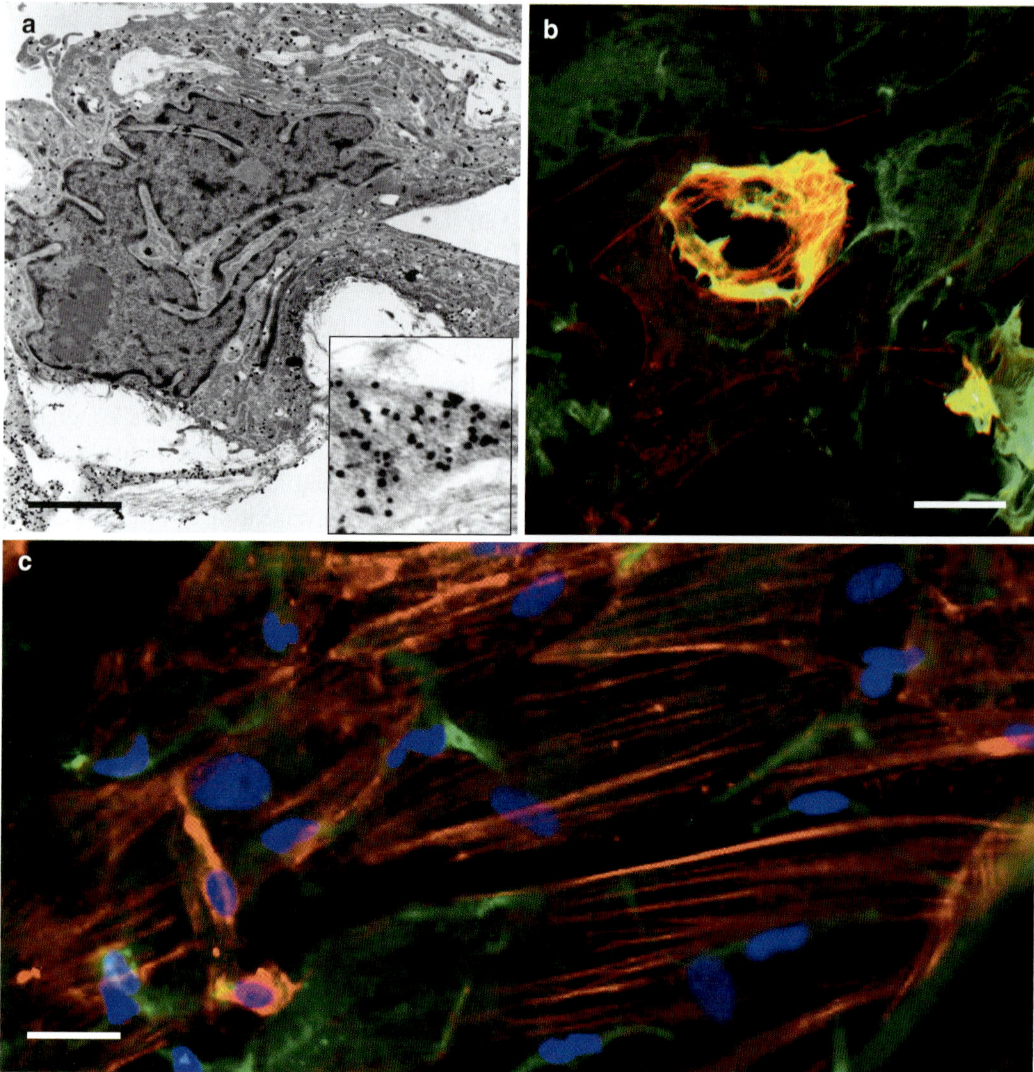

Fig. 5.3 Cellular elements of contraction in epiretinal membranes. Transmission electron micrograph presents (**a**) an ultrathin section after pre-embedding preparation of internal limiting membrane (ILM) specimen with epiretinal cell proliferation allowing for ultrastructural and immunocytochemical characterisation of cellular elements. Myofibroblasts were identified by positive labelling with immunonanogold particles (insert) against α-smooth muscle actin (α-SMA) filaments. Fluorescence micrographs (**b**, **c**) demonstrate flat-mounted ILM specimens with epiretinal cell proliferation that were double labelled for anti-α-SMA (*red*) and anti-vimentin (*green*) in addition to cell nuclei staining (*blue*) by 4′,6-diamidino-2-phenylindole (DAPI). Co-localisation (*yellow*) of α-SMA and vimentin is presented by a subpopulation of myofibroblasts only (Specimens were surgically removed during vitrectomy from eyes with macular pucker and macular holes at the Department of Ophthalmology, Ludwig-Maximilians-University Munich, Germany. Original magnification: (a) ×4,800, scale bar=2.1 μm; (b) ×20, scale bar=500 μm; (c) ×40, scale bar=250 μm)

and Ishibashi 2011; Kohno et al. 2009; Hirayama et al. 2004). Since immunoreactivity for α-SMA was even found in hypocellular membranes of macular traction disorders, transdifferentiation of epiretinal cells into myofibroblasts appears to occur early in the disease development (Schumann et al. 2011). Presumably both glial cells and hyalocytes are potent candidates to generate epiretinal membrane contraction by myofibroblast-like transdifferentiation.

Conclusion

Persistent vitreo-macular adhesions, vitreoschisis with cortical vitreous remnants on the ILM and epiretinal fibrocellular proliferation are associated with vitreo-macular traction. Whereas age-related PVD is generally accepted as an important pathogenic factor in the development of vitreo-macular traction, the significance of cellular proliferation and migration is still under debate. In the light of the current literature and in our own experience, epiretinal cell proliferations are an essential part of the pathophysiology of vitreo-macular traction by anchoring vitreo-macular adhesions to the retina, thereby tightening the vitreoretinal juncture and transmitting dynamic traction forces in the long term. Both hyalocyte activation in the vitreous cortex and glial cell activation in retinal layers appear to be initiated by age-related vitreous changes driving cell mediated traction at the vitreoretinal interface as a prerequisite for the development of vitreo-macular traction disorders.

Compliance with Ethical Requirements Dr Gandorfer is a consultant for Thrombogenics, Alcon, Santen, Oertli. Dr Schumann has no conflicts of interest. No animal or human studies were carried out by the authors for this chapter.

Acknowledgements We are especially grateful to Anselm Kampik, Professor and Chairman of the Department of Ophthalmology at the Ludwig-Maximilians-University Munich, for his enduring support and contribution to our studies. We also would like to thank Christos Haritoglou for his dedication and continuing collaboration. Regarding electron microscopy, we would like to thank Renate Scheler, Helga Wehnes and Axel K. Walch for their outstanding technical assistance.

References

Balazs EA, Toth LZ, Eckl EA et al (1964) Studies on the structure of the vitreous body. XII. Cytologicall and histochemical studies on the cortical tissue layer. Exp Eye Res 3:57–71

Bando H, Ikuno Y, Choi JS et al (2005) Ultrastructure of internal limiting membrane in myopic foveoschisis. Am J Ophthalmol 391:197–199

Bishop PN, Holmes DF, Kadler KE et al (2004) Age-related changes on the surface of the vitreous collagen fibrils. Invest Ophthalmol Vis Sci 45:1041–1046

Bringmann A, Wiedemann P (2009) Involvement of Müller glial cells in epiretinal membrane formation. Graefes Arch Clin Exp Ophthalmol 247:865–883

Bringmann A, Pannicke T, Grosche J et al (2006) Müller cells in the healthy and diseased retina. Prog Retin Eye Res 25:397–424

Dallon JC, Ehrlich HP (2010) Differences in the mechanism of collagen lattice contraction by myofibroblasts and smooth muscle cells. J Cell Biochem 111:362–369

Dingemans KP, Teeling P (1994) Long-spacing collagen and proteoglycans in pathologic tissue. Ultrastruct Pathol 18:539–547

Eyden A, Tzaphlidou M (2001) Structural variants of collagen in normal and pathologic tissues: role of electron microscopy. Micron 32:287–300

Fekrat S, Wendel RT, de la Cruz Z et al (1995) Clinicopathologic correlation of an epiretinal membrane associated with a recurrent macular hole. Retina 15:53–57

Fisher SK, Lewis GP (2003) Müller cell and neuronal remodeling in retinal attachment and reattachment and their potential consequences for visual recovery: a review and reconsideration of recent data. Vision Res 43:887–897

Gandorfer A (2007) Diffuse diabetic macular edema: pathology and implications for surgery. Dev Ophthalmol 39:88–95

Gandorfer A (2009) Objective of pharmacologic vitreolysis. Dev Ophthalmol 44:1–6

Gandorfer A, Rohleder M, Kampik A (2002) Epiretinal pathology of vitreomacular traction syndrome. Br J Ophthalmol 86:902–909

Gandorfer A, Rohleder M, Grosselfinger S et al (2005) Epiretinal pathology of diffuse diabetic macular edema associated with vitreomacular traction. Am J Ophthalmol 139:638–652

Gandorfer A, Scheler R, Schumann R et al (2009) Interference microscopy delineates cellular proliferations on flat mounted internal limiting membrane specimens. Br J Ophthalmol 93:120–122

Gandorfer A, Schumann R, Scheler R et al (2011) Pores of the inner limiting membrane in flat-mounted surgical specimens. Retina 31:977–981

Gandorfer A, Haritoglou C, Scheler R et al (2012) Residual cellular proliferation on the internal limting membrane in macular pucker surgery. Retina 32(3):477–485, [Epub ahead of print]. PMID: 22068175

Gastaud P, Bétis F, Rouhette H et al (2000) Ultrastructural findings of epimacular membrane and detached posterior hyaloid in vitreomacular traction syndrome. J Fr Ophtalmol 23:587–593

Green WR (2006) The macular hole: histopathologic studies. Arch Ophthalmol 124:317–321

Grierson I, Mazure A, Hogg P et al (1996) Non-vascular vitreoretinopathy: the cells and the cellular basis of contraction. Eye 10:671–684

Gupta P, Yee KM, Garcia P et al (2011) Vitreoschisis in macular diseases. Br J Ophthalmol 95:376–380

Hannover A (1845) Entdeckung des Baues des Glaskörpers. Müller Arch 467–477

Haritoglou C, Schumann RG, Kampik A et al (2007) Glial cell proliferation under the internal limiting membrane in a patient with cellophane maculopathy. Arch Ophthalmol 125:1301–1302

Heidenkummer HP, Kampik A (1992) Proliferative activity and immunohistochemical cell differentiation in human epiretinal membranes. Ger J Ophthalmol 1:170–175

Hirayama K, Hata Y, Noda Y et al (2004) The involvement of the rho-kinase pathway and its regulation in cytokine-induced collagen gel contraction by hyalocytes. Invest Ophthalmol Vis Sci 45:3896–3903

Hiscott PS, Grierson I, McLeod D (1984a) Retinal pigment epithelial cells in epiretinal membranes: an immunohistochemical study. Br J Ophthalmol 68:708–715

Hiscott PS, Grierson I, Trombetta CJ et al (1984b) Retinal and epiretinal glia – an immunochistochemical study. Br J Ophthalmol 68:698–707

Ishida S, Yamazaki K, Shinoda K et al (2000) Macular hole retinal detachment in highly myopic eyes. Ultrastructure of surgically removed epiretinal membrane and clinicopathologic correlation. Retina 20:176–183

Johnson MW (2002) Improvements in the understanding and treatment of macular hole. Curr Opin Ophthalmol 13:152–160

Johnson MW (2005a) Perifoveal vitreous detachment and its macular complications. Trans Am Ophthalmol Soc 103:537–567

Johnson MW (2005b) Tractional cystoid macular edema: a subtle variant of the vitreomacular traction syndrome. Am J Ophthalmol 140:184–192

Johnson MW (2009) Etiology and treatment of macular edema. Am J Ophthalmol 147:11–21

Johnson MW (2010) Posterior vitreous detachment: evolution and complications of its early stages. Am J Ophthalmol 49:371–382

Kampik A, Green WR, Michels RG et al (1980) Ultrastructural features of progressive idiopathic epiretinal membrane removed by vitreous surgery. Am J Ophthalmol 90:797–809

Kampik A, Kenyon KB, Michels RG et al (1981) Epiretinal and vitreous membranes: comparative study of 56 cases. Arch Ophthalmol 99:1445–1454

Kenawy N, Wong D, Stappler T et al (2010) Does the presence of an epiretinal membrane alter the retinal cleavage plan during internal limiting membrane peeling? Ophthalmology 117:320–323

Kodal H, Weick M, Moll V et al (2000) Involvement of calcium-activated potassium channels in the regulation of DNA synthesis in cultured Müller glial cells. Invest Ophthalmol Vis Sci 41:4262–4267

Kohno T, Sorgnte N, Ishibashi T et al (1987) Immunofluorescence studies of fibronectin and laminin in the human eye. Invest Ophthalmol Vis Sci 28:500–514

Kohno RI, Hata Y, Kawahara S et al (2009) Possible contribution of hyalocytes to idiopathic epiretinal membrane formation and its contraction. Br J Ophthalmol 93:1020–1026

Krebs I, Brannath W, Glittenberg C et al (2007) Posterior vitreomacular adhesion: a potential risk factor for exudative age-related macular degeneration. Am J Ophthalmol 144:741–746

Krebs I, Glittenberg C, Zeiler F, Binder S (2011) Spectral domain optical coherence tomography for higher precision in the evaluation of vitreoretinal adhesions in exudative age-related macular degeneration. Br J Ophthalmol 95:1415–1418

Lazarus HS, Hageman GS (1994) In situ characterization of the human hyalocytes. Arch Ophthalmol 112:1356–1362

Lesnik Oberstein SY, Lewis GP, Dutra T et al (2011) Evidence that neurites in human epiretinal membranes express melanopsin, calretinin, rodopsin and neurofilament protein. Br J Ophthalmol 95:266–272

Lewis GP, Fisher SK (2003) Up-regulation of glial fibrillary acidic protein in response to retinal injury: its potential role in glial remodeling and a comparison to vimentin expression. Int Rev Cytol 230:263–290

Lindqvist N, Liu Q, Zajadacz J et al (2010) Retinal glial (Müller) cells: sensing and responding to tissue stretch. Invest Ophthalmol Vis Sci 51:1683–1690

Messmer EM, Heidenkummer HP, Kampik A (1998) Ultrastructure of epiretinal membranes associated with macular holes. Graefes Arch Clin Exp Ophthalmol 236:248–254

Nakazawa T, Takeda M, Lewis GP et al (2007) Attenuated glial reactions and photoreceptor degeneration after retinal detachment in mice deficient in glial fibrillary acidic protein and vimentin. Invest Ophthalmol Vis Sci 48:2760–2768

Parolini B, Schumann RG, Cereda MM et al (2011) Lamellar macular hole: a clinicopathologic correlation of surgically excised internal limiting membrane specimens. Invest Ophthalmol Vis Sci 52:9074–9083

Qiao H, Hisatomi T, Sonoda KH et al (2005) The characterisation of hyalocytes: the origin, phenotype, and turnover. Br J Ophthalmol 89:513–517

Russel SR, Shepherd JD, Hageman GS (1991) Distribution of glycoconjugates in the human retinal internal limiting membrane. Invest Ophthalmol Vis Sci 32:1986–1995

Sakamoto T, Ishibashi T (2011) Hyalocytes: essential cells of the vitreous cavity in vitreoretinal pathophysiology? Retina 31:222–228

Schumann RG, Gandorfer A (2010) Vitreoretinal degenerative macular diseases. Klin Monbl Augenheilkd 227:R49–R60

Schumann RG, Schaumberger M, Rohleder M et al (2006) Ultrastructure of the vitromacular interface in full-thickness idiopathic macular holes: a consecutive analysis of 100 cases. Am J Ophthalmol 141:1112–1119

Schumann RG, Schaumberger MM, Rohleder M et al (2007) The primary objective in macular hole surgery. Ultrastructural features of the vitreomacular interface. Ophthalmologe 104:783–789

Schumann RG, Rohleder M, Schaumberger MM et al (2008) Idiopathic macular holes: ultrastructural aspects of surgical failure. Retina 28:340–349

Schumann RG, Eibl KH, Zhao F et al (2011) Immunocytochemical and ultrastructural evidence of glial cells and hyalocytes in internal limiting membrane specimens of idiopathic macular holes. Invest Ophthalmol Vis Sci 3:7822–7834

Schwartz SD, Alexander R, Hiscott P et al (1996) Recognition of vitreoschisis in proliferative diabetic retinopathy. A useful landmark in vitrectomy for diabetic traction retinal detachment. Ophthalmology 103:323–328

Sebag J (1996) Diabetic vitreopathy. Ophthalmology 103:205–206

Sebag J (2004) Anomalous posterior vitreous detachment: a unifying concept in vitreo-retinal disease. Graefes Arch Clin Exp Ophthalmol 242:690–698

Sebag J (2008) Vitreochisis. Graefes Arch Clin Exp Ophthalmol 246:329–332

Sebag J, Gupta P, Rosen RR et al (2007) Macular holes and macular pucker: the role of vitreoschisis as imaged by optical coherence tomography/scanning laser ophthalmoscopy. Trans Am Ophthalmol Soc 105:121–129

Sebag J, Wang MY, Nguyen D et al (2009) Vitreopapillary adhesion in macular diseases. Trans Am Ophthalmol Soc 107:35–46

Shinoda K, Hirakata A, Hida T et al (2000) Ultrastructural and immunohistochemical findings in five patients with vitreomacular traction syndrome. Retina 20:289–293

Smiddy WE, Maguire AM, Green WR et al (1989) Idiopathic epiretinal membranes: ultrastructural characteristics and clinicopathologic correlation. Ophthalmology 96:811–820

Uchino E, Uemura A, Ohba N (2001) Initial stages of posterior vitreous detachment in healthy eyes of older persons evaluated by optical coherence tomography. Arch Ophthalmol 119:1475–1479

Vanderbeek BL, Johnson MW (2012) The diversity of traction mechanisms in myopic traction maculopathy. Am J Ophthalmol 153:93–102

Vinores SA, Campochiaro PA, Conway BP (1990) Ultrastructural and electron-immunocytochemical characterization of cells in epiretinal membranes. Invest Ophthalmol Vis Sci 31:14–28

Yoshida M, Kishi S (2007) Pathogenesis of macular hole recurrence and its prevention by internal limiting membrane peeling. Retina 27:169–173

Imaging of the Vitreo-macular Interface

6

Carl Glittenberg and Susanne Binder

6.1 Introduction

The necessity for an effective and clinically efficient method for imaging and documenting subtle physiological and pathological structures of the vitreo-retinal interface is becoming increasingly evident. Other than the direct mechanical effects of vitreo-retinal traction, several studies have shown the correlation between vitreo-retinal adhesion and the presence of AMD (Krebs et al. 2011). With the advent of vitreolytic pharmacological injections into the eye (Girach A et al. 2012), it is pivotal to be able to not only use imaging to ascertain which patients would benefit from treatment but also to objectively document the effect of the treatment on the vitreous.

Although there are several methods and technologies that can be used to image the vitreous *in vitro* and *in vivo* (Sebag 2004), only clinically relevant techniques to image the vitreous *in vivo* will be discussed in this chapter. Both biomicroscopy and ultrasound are important methods of imaging the vitreous, but their usefulness in imaging the actual vitreo-retinal interface is limited. Ultrasound will be briefly discussed, but the main focus of this chapter will be on optical coherence technology (OCT) imaging, as this technology is rapidly becoming the imaging modality of choice due to its speed, resolution, reproducibility, and noninvasiveness.

Different OCT noise reduction methods as well as three-dimensional visualization systems will be discussed. The benefit of virtual en face C-scans will be presented. At the end of this chapter, a short description of intraoperative OCT visualization will be provided.

6.2 Ultrasound

Due to the relatively low resolution and the focus of the technology on the vitreous core (Sebag 2004), the importance of ultrasound in imaging the vitreo-retinal interface has been steadily decreasing since the advent of Fourier domain OCT. Additionally, the necessity of contact between the corneal surface and the ultrasound instrument probe results in an examination method, which is uncomfortable for the patient and potentially a source of mechanical trauma and infection. In contrast, OCT examination, being a noncontact procedure, has virtually no risk of trauma and has a greatly reduced risk of infection. As a correctly performed ultrasound examination of the vitreo-retinal interface requires not only a skilled examiner but also a complaint patient and significant amount of time, OCT examinations have largely replaced ultrasound examinations, except for patients with opaque media.

C. Glittenberg, MD (✉) • S. Binder, MD
Department of Ophthalmology,
Ludwig Boltzmann Institute for Retinology
and Biomicroscopic Laser Surgery,
Rudolf Foundation Hospital,
Juchgasse 25, 1030 Vienna, Austria
e-mail: carl.glittenberg@wienkav.at

A. Girach, M.D. de Smet (eds.), *Diseases of the Vitreo-Macular Interface*, Essentials in Ophthalmology,
DOI 10.1007/978-3-642-40034-6_6, © Springer-Verlag Berlin Heidelberg 2014

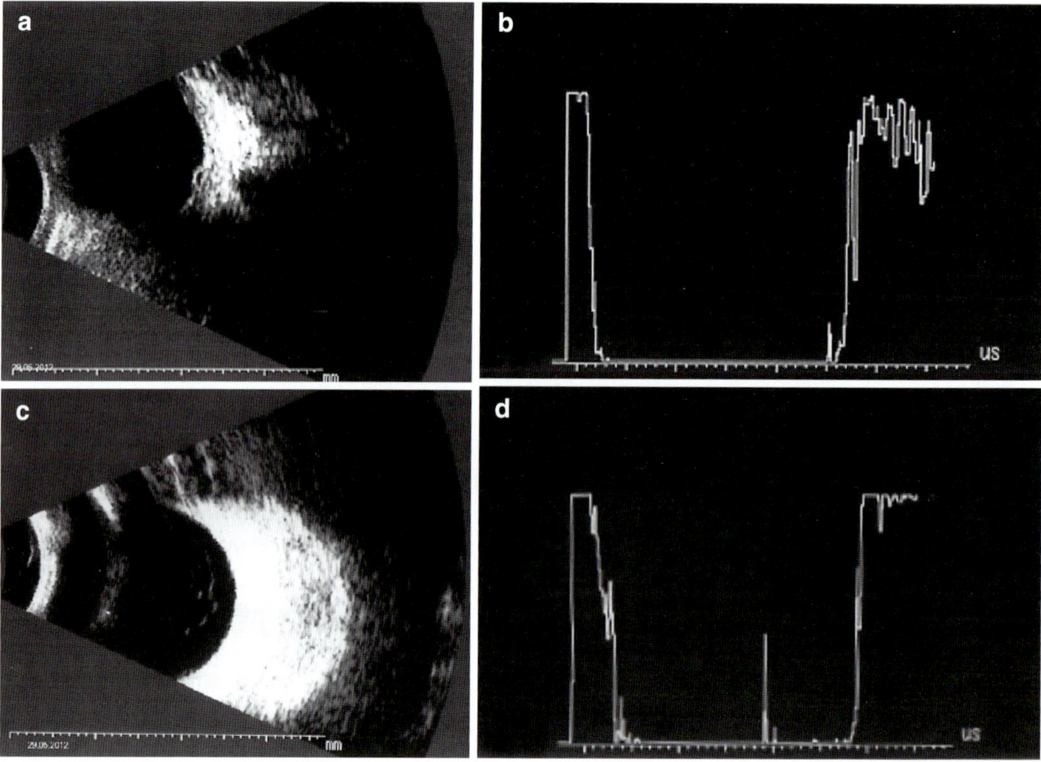

Fig. 6.1 10 MHZ retinal ultrasound images. *Top*: B-mode and A-mode scans of a pigment epithelium detachment. *Bottom*: B-mode and A-mode scans of a complete detachment of the posterior vitreous

Ultrasound does however remain an indispensible tool when ascertaining whether the vitreous is completely attached or completely detached from the retina. At this time, commercially available OCT software and hardware are not able distinguish between completely attached posterior vitreous structures and the surface of the retina (Krebs et al. 2011). Unless one has access to a previous OCT examination of the same patient, in which a partial vitreous detachment is visible, it is not possible to determine whether a vitreous that is not visible in the OCT is completely attached or completely detached and located above the scan depth of the OCT, which is typically approximately 2,000 µm (see Fig. 6.1).

The second considerable drawback of ultrasound in comparison to modern OCT technology is the lower resolution. Where a typical, commercially available, Fourier domain OCT has an axial resolution of approximately 5 µm, the axial resolution of a 10 MHZ ultrasound is approximately 150 µm (Drexler 2004). An ultrasound with a high-frequency transducer (50 MHZ) can achieve an axial resolution of 20–30 µm, but this comes at the cost reducing the tissue penetration to 4 mm, making it useful only for imaging the anterior chamber and not the retina (Drexler 2004).

6.3 OCT

Since the first appearance of a commercially available OCT onto the ophthalmic market in 1996 (Drexler 2004), OCT technology has been steadily taking over as the most important modality for retinal imaging. The first two generations of ophthalmic OCT systems did not have the resolution or speed necessary to make them clinically useful for identifying subtle changes in the vitreo-retinal interface. Even the third-generation Stratus OCT™, which already had an axial resolution of 10 µm, was a time domain-based system which had a high signal-to-noise ratio to pick up vitreous structures reliably. First the development of an ophthalmic Fourier domain OCT (Wojtkowski et al. 2001) in 2001 heralded a revolution in the field of vitreo-retinal interface imaging. Over the last 10 years, the speed and imaging quality of commercially available OCT has made several quantum leaps.

Currently there are over half a dozen commercially available Fourier domain OCTs on the market. They all have an approximate axial resolution of between 5 and 7 µm and a lateral resolution of about 14–20 µm. Typical single B-mode scans will be about 6–9 mm wide and 2 mm deep. In this chapter we will be focusing on the capabilities of the Heidelberg Engineering™ Spectralis OCT™ and the Carl Zeiss Meditec™ Cirrus HD-OCT™ 4000. Most commercially available systems have similar capabilities to these two systems. Therefore, the topics discussed in this chapter will pertain to other systems as well.

In the last decade Fourier domain OCT has established itself as the prime imaging modality for vitreo-macular traction syndrome, cystoid macular edema/diabetic macular edema, epiretinal membranes, full-thickness macular holes, and schisis (Mirza et al. 2007). Please see Fig. 6.2 for some examples of the types of images of these pathologies that can be obtained with a modern OCT. Details to the pathologies themselves have been provided in previous chapters of this book. Please note the ability of the OCT to visualize subtle vitreal structures like the remnants of Cloquet's channel and vitreo-schisis in Fig. 6.2a. In order to obtain the type of high-quality images that can be seen in Figs. 6.2 and 6.4, it is necessary to increase the signal-to-noise ratio of the raw OCT data. This subject is covered in the next section.

6.3.1 Noise Reduction

One of the biggest problems with raw OCT data when trying to visualize the vitreous and the vitreo-retinal interface is differentiating actual vitreous structure from background noise. For this reason most modern OCT systems have the ability to perform a noise reduction during post processing. Figure 6.3 shows a scan in three different stages of noise reduction. Such noise reduction can be achieved in fundamentally two different ways.

On one hand one can use a tracked OCT system like the Spectralis OCT™, which is able to repeat the OCT scan in exactly the same place several times and then average the resulting images (Fig. 6.4). The amount of repeated and averaged images can be set to between two images and over 100 images. This has the benefit that it creates some stunning results and can be repeated at exactly the same location during a follow-up examination. The drawback is that it is very time consuming during acquisition time.

The other alternative, the method used by the Cirrus HD-OCT, is to perform noise reduction algorithms in post processing without the need for tracking (Fig. 6.3). The Cirrus HD-OCT™ allows two settings for the oversampling. In the first setting the instrument will take a raster of five HD scans and perform an internal oversampling of these images. This is possible because the size of the raw data of an OCT scan is approximately 4 times wider in pixels than the optical resolution allows. In other words, the instrument will acquire 4 lateral pixels per unit of resolution. This is down sampled during display. These pixels can however be used to differentiate noise from signal, resulting in an image that is oversampled 4 times (Fig. 6.4 middle). In the second mode, all five scans are almost simultaneously acquired from the same position of the retina and a composite image created through a selective pixel profiling algorithm, resulting in a single image that is oversampled 20 times (Fig. 6.4 bottom). This does not create quite as stunning images and does not give one the possibility to repeat the scan in exactly the same place during a follow-up examination, but has the benefit of being considerably faster during acquisition time, posing a smaller burden on the patient.

Which system is clinically more useful is largely a matter opinion. It should be mentioned however that the Cirrus HD-OCT™ can only perform this type of noise reduction on 5-line or single-line HD scans and not on three-dimensional cubes. The Spectralis OCT™ can perform the

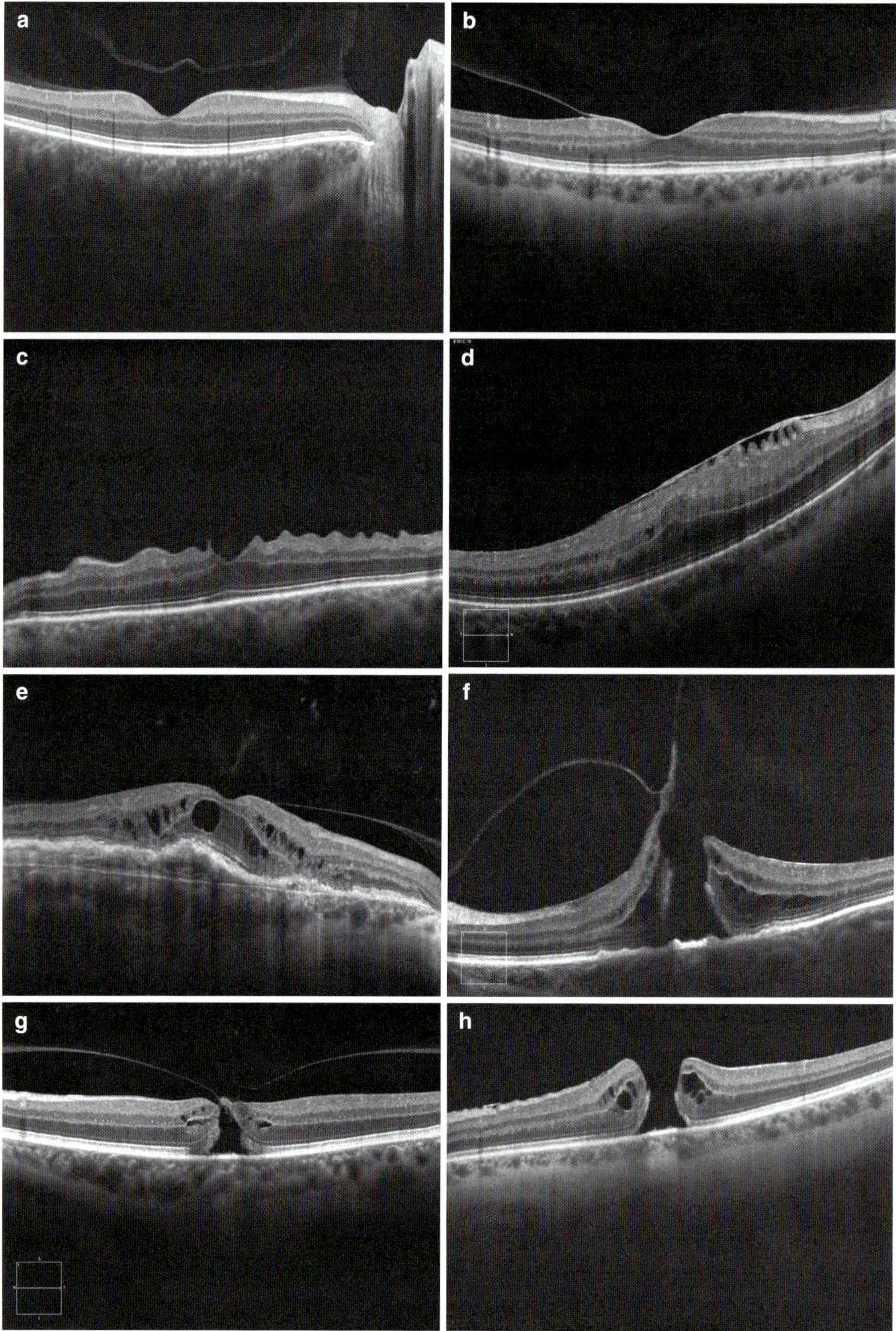

Fig. 6.2 Cirrus HD-OCT™ HD scans (20 times oversampling): (**a**) vitreo-schisis; (**b**) vitreo-macular traction; (**c**) macular pucker; (**d**) epiretinal membrane; (**e**) CNV with vitreo-macular traction; (**f**) vitreo-retinal traction with macular hole; (**g**) vitreo-retinal traction with macular hole; (**h**) macular hole

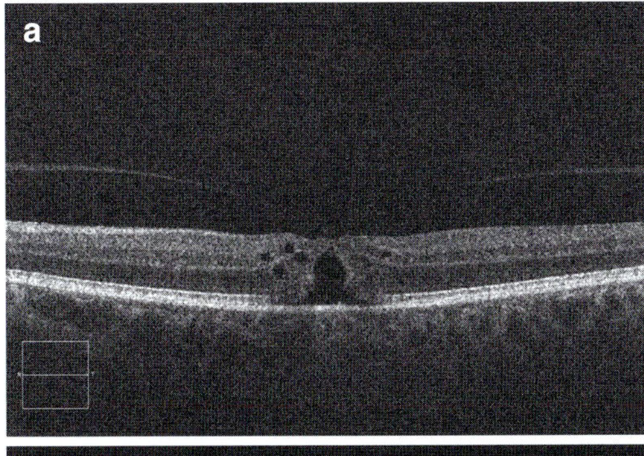

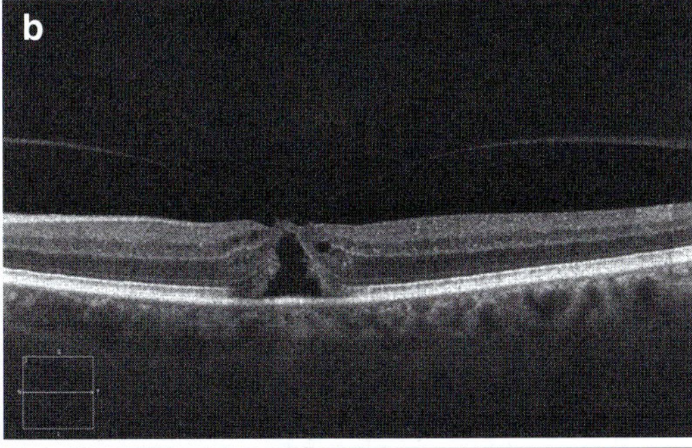

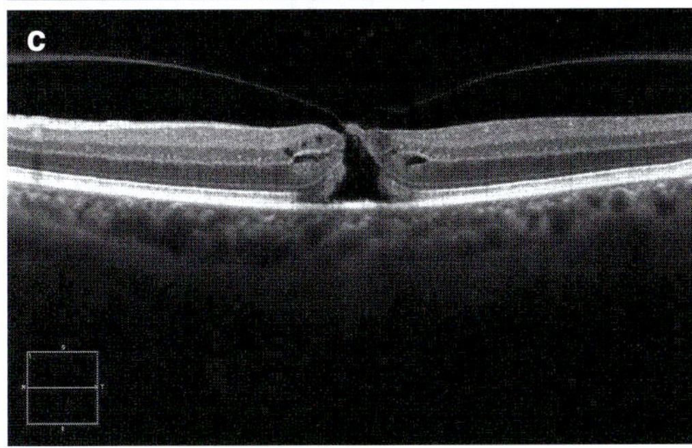

Fig. 6.3 Cirrus HD-OCT™ HD scans: (**a**) no oversampling; (**b**) 4 times oversampling; (**c**): 20 times oversampling

averaging on an entire cube, but the acquisition time quickly becomes prohibitively long.

6.3.2 ILM Segmentation

It is important to point out that although most OCT software claim to have the ability to create a segmentation layer of the internal limiting membrane (ILM), this statement is very misleading. The software algorithms will recognize, with varying degrees of accuracy, the retinal surface or more specifically the change in intensity of the reflection of the scanning beam as it passes from vitreous (or fluid) into the retina. This resulting interface will then be segmented into the so-called ILM layer. In patients that have not had vitreo-retinal surgery including membrane peeling, this difference is irrelevant, but in patients that have had surgery, the algorithms are not able to differentiate whether the ILM has been removed or not. These algorithms are not particularly useful when it comes to visualizing or quantifying the vitreo-retinal interface but are rather used to calculate retinal thickness and volume. They can be very useful in quantifying changes in retinal thickness due to disease or therapy.

6.3.3 RPE-Fit Slab Visualization

Although this section describes a method using a software feature primarily available on the

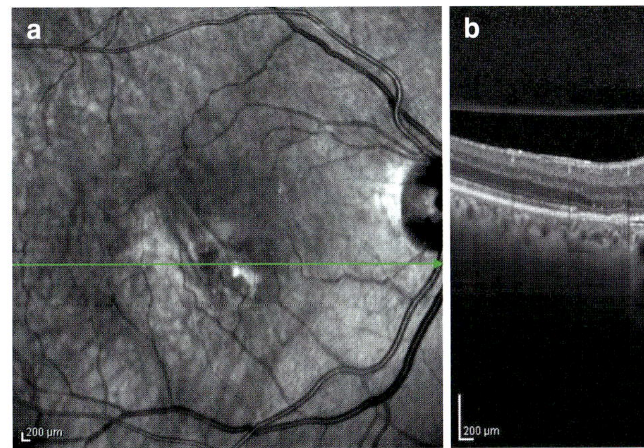

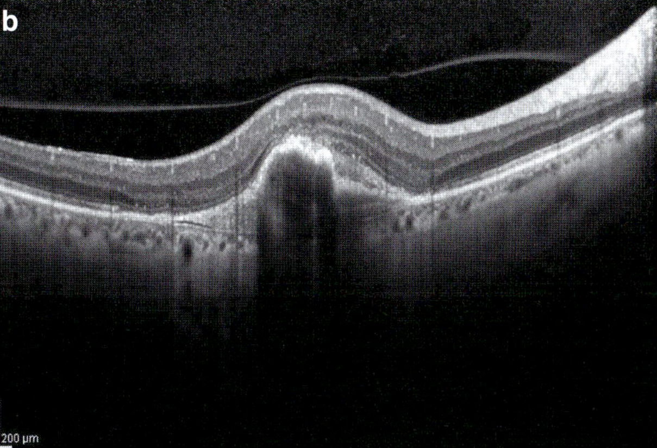

Fig. 6.4 Spectralis OCT™ of AMD and a PVD (no traction) with 36 times averaging

Carl Zeiss Meditec™ Cirrus HD-OCT™, the concept is applicable to any commercial OCT system, provided the scan pattern is dense enough. The Cirrus HD-OCT™ typically creates a macular cube scan of 128 scans. Each scan has $512 \times 1{,}024$ pixels. The area of the scan is 6×6 mm. If the resulting cube is cut at any given height, one receives a virtual en face C-scan with an area of 6×6 mm and a resolution of 46.9 µm in the y-axis (distance between B-mode scans) and 15 µm (transverse resolution) in the x-axis.

A strictly horizontal slice through the cube is noted to be useful, which is why it is possible to create an "RPE-fit" slab (see Fig. 6.5). The thickness of this slab can be set by the user, but a setting of approximately 100 µm has proven useful for most situations. The contour of the slab is automatically set to follow the contour of the RPE. The height of the slab can be set at any given position, so that it is possible to scroll through the retinal structures from the vitreo-retinal interface to the choroid while maintaining an overview of the relative positions of all structures.

The usefulness of this method is illustrated in Fig. 6.5. It shows the case of a patient with a vitreo-retinal tractive adhesion and a CNV. In order to visualize the spatial correlation between the tangential tractions, the point of adhesion, and the location of the CNV, a 100 µm, "RPE-fit" slab was slowly panned through the structures along the z-axis. The spatial correlation was thus clearly demonstrated. More details to the correlation of vitreo-retinal adhesion and AMD can be found in a previous chapter.

Such visualization could of course have been done with a strictly horizontal en face image, but to have the virtual C-scan adjust itself, the curvature of the retinal structures improves the continuity of the structural visualization.

This type of visualization can of course only be performed on data that has a dense enough scan pattern. On the Spectralis™ OCT the scan density should therefore be increased to over 100 to get a similar result.

6.3.4 Commercial 3D Visualization

There are essentially two different methods of displaying three-dimensional data that are used by the currently commercially available OCT systems. On one hand one has the method used by, for example, the Spectralis OCT™, which essentially projects B-mode scans on a topology of the retina (Fig. 6.6 top). This has the benefit that it creates very crisp visualizations at the cost of removing the vitreous from the image. The second method is the one used by the Cirrus HD-OCT™ (Fig. 6.6 bottom) which creates 3D visualizations that can show the structures of the vitreous but are hazy and indistinct due to the low signal-to-noise ratio. Both types have the benefit that they can be rendered in real time. The clinical and scientific usefulness of 3D visualizations has been very limited as there did not seem to be any additional information in the 3D visualization that could not be gained from simply scrolling through the B-mode scans.

6.3.5 Experimental 3D Visualization

Although the clinical relevance of 3D OCT visualization has been low, attempts have been made to create new algorithms that show subtle 3D structures in a more useful way. Already in 2007 the advantages of a ray-traced 3D rendering system were demonstrated (Glittenberg et al. 2009). Figure 6.7 shows several 3D visualizations of vitreo-retinal structures using a derivative algorithm of the one originally presented in 2007. This visualization system, in comparison to conventional systems, calculates ray-traced shading, resulting in a greatly enhanced 3D contrast. Additionally several noise reduction algorithms have been implemented to heighten the visibility of subtle structures inside the vitreous.

On the top two images of Fig. 6.7, one sees a patient with vitreo-schisis. The left image shows the visualization with a high noise cutoff level effectively removing vitreous structures. The

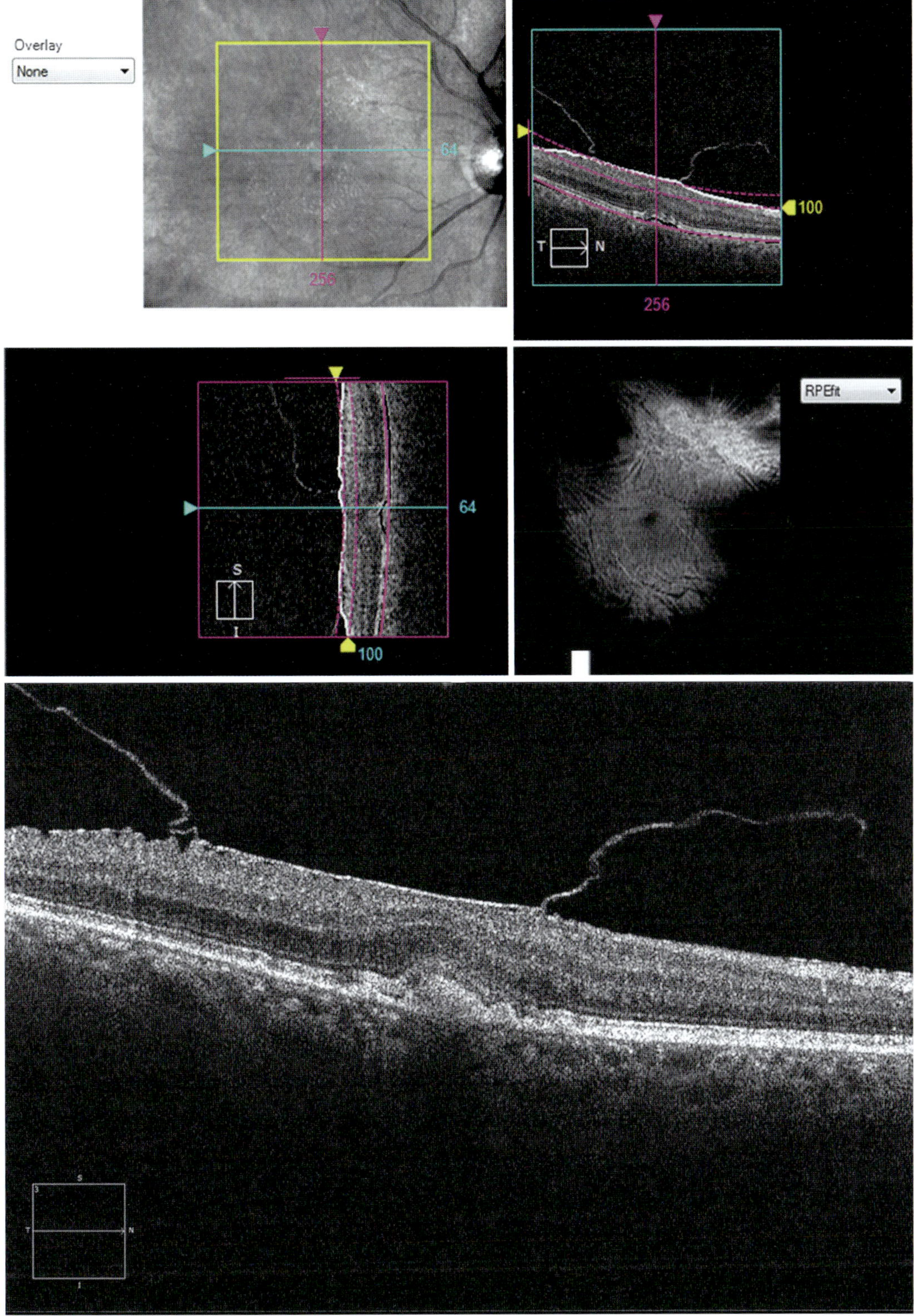

Fig. 6.5 Cirrus HD-OCT™ RPE-fit virtual en face C-scans of a patient with vitreo-retinal tractive adhesion and CNV

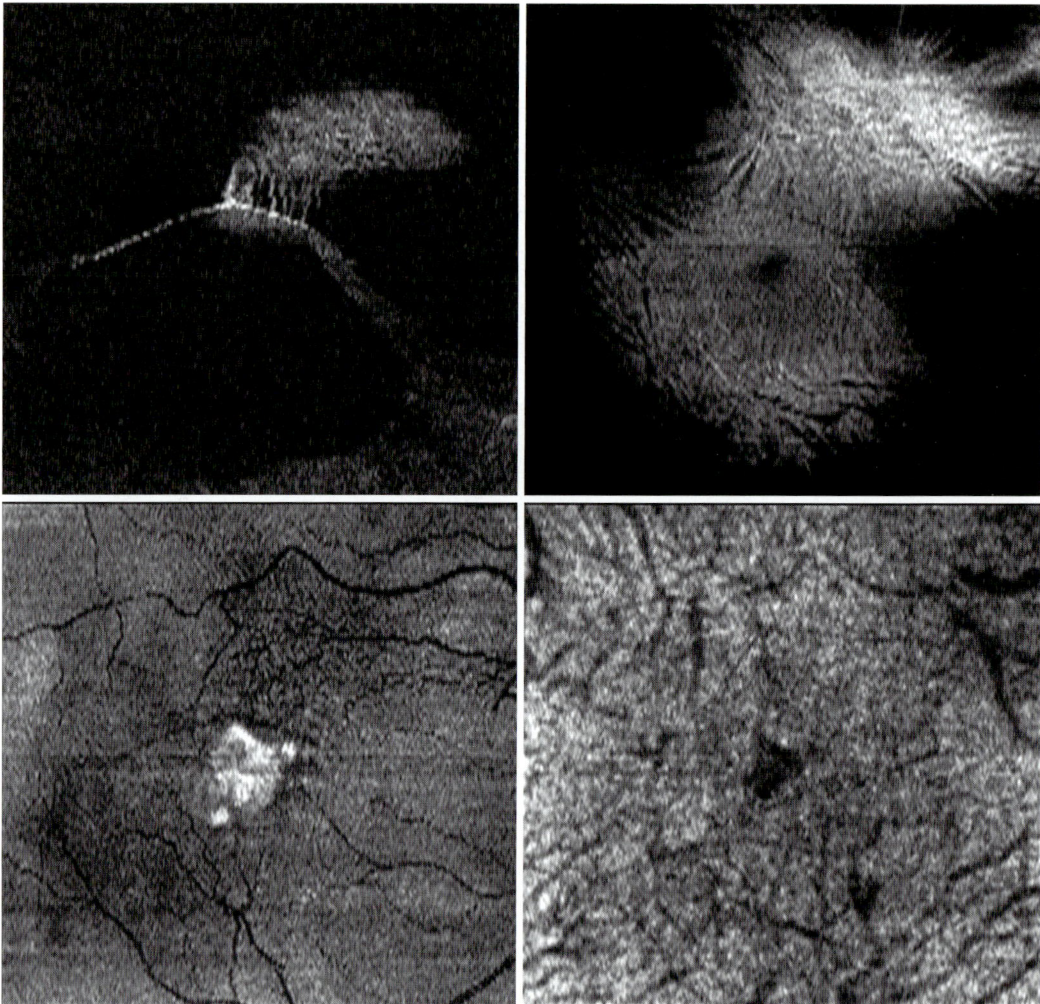

Fig. 6.5 (continued)

right image shows the same patient with lower noise cutoff level. As the data has been through the new noise reduction algorithms, the vitreo-schisis becomes visible in the area around the optic nerve head. The two middle images of Fig. 6.7 show a patient with vitreo-macular traction. Due to the nature of the visualization system, the areas of attachment can be clearly differentiated. The bottom two images in Fig. 6.8 show a patient with a vitreo-retinal adhesion and a CNV. The 3D visualization helps clarify the correlation between location of the adhesion and the location of the CNV. More specifically the 3D visualization shows that the CNV lies at the intersection point of the tangential traction lines of the adhesion.

With the correlation between vitreo-retinal traction and AMD becoming more evident (Krebs et al. 2011) and vitreolytic therapies becoming available (Girach et al. 2012), such a method of visualization will become critical for efficacy studies and clinical diagnosis as well as follow-up.

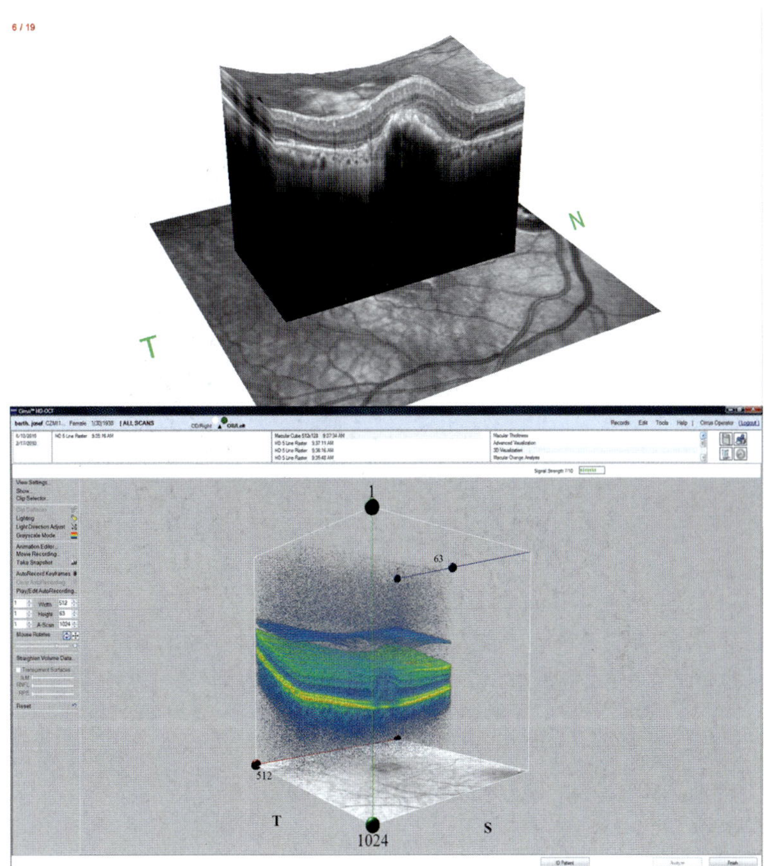

Fig. 6.6 Commercial 3D visualization systems: *top*: Spectralis OCT™; *bottom*: Cirrus HD-OCT™

6.4 Intrasurgical OCT

The last several years have shown the emergence of intraoperative OCT visualization (Binder et al. 2011; Hahn et al. 2013). At this time these systems still only exist as prototypes, but should be mentioned, as they will play an increasingly important role in surgical retina in the future. In these systems the OCT scanning module is placed directly in the optical pathway of the surgical microscope allowing a live OCT recording of the surgical procedure. High-definition scans, 3D cubes, and layer segmentations are also possible with these systems. As the signal-to-noise ratio in these systems tends to be fairly high in comparison to conventional OCTs, methods of enhancing the visibility of the vitreous are being developed. One of these methods (Glittenberg et al. 2012) is the injection of triamcinolone acetate after the core vitrectomy in order to visualize the remnants of the posterior vitreous (Fig. 6.8). Triamcinolone was used as its crystalline structure manages to scatter a part of the beam without obscuring structures under it. It was also chosen because it is not retinotoxic and has already been approved for intrasurgical use. With this visualization system it may be possible to get a better understanding of the mechanical dynamics of vitreo-retinal adhesions during removal.

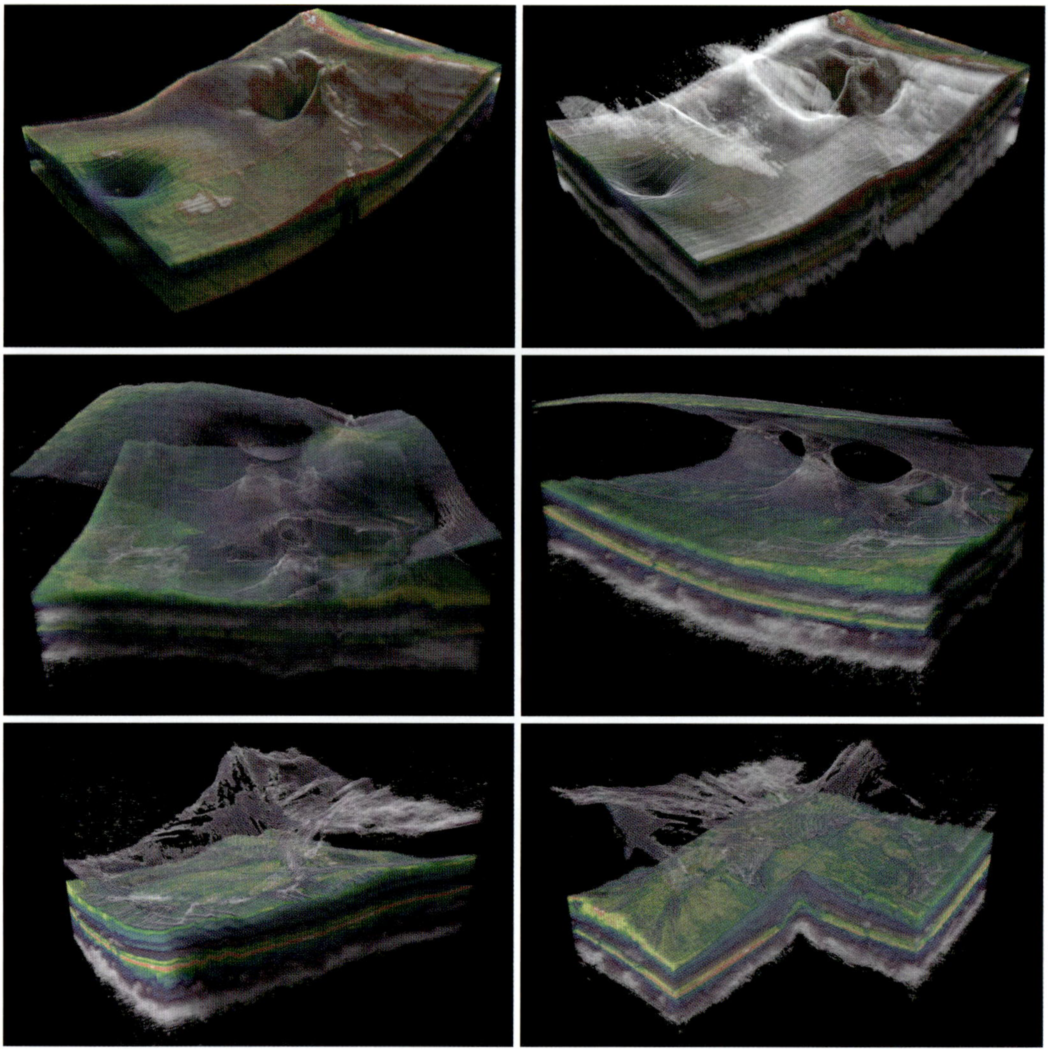

Fig. 6.7 Prototype ray-traced 3D visualization system: *top*: vitreo-schisis; *middle*: vitreo-retinal traction; *bottom*: vitreo-retinal adhesion with CNV

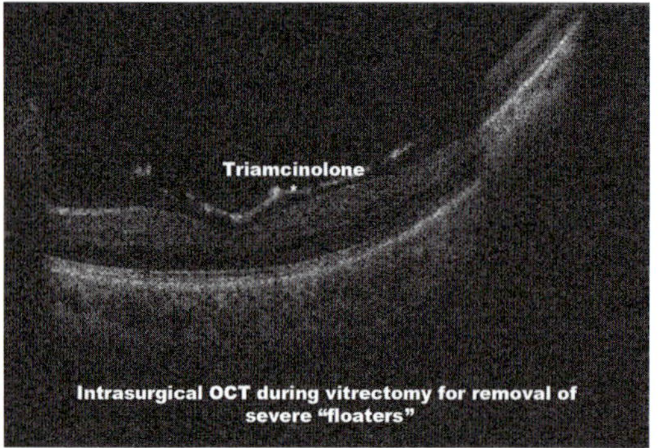

Fig. 6.8 Triamcinolone contrast enhancement of the posterior vitreous in an intraoperative OCT during vitrectomy

Conclusion

The future of imaging of the vitreo-retinal interface lies in the next developments in OCT technology. In the next years we will see a significant increase in scan density as well as scan speed. This will result in instruments being able to create a $512 \times 512 \times 1{,}024$ macular cube in half the time that it takes now. Additionally these scans will be able to encompass a much larger area of the fundus in a single acquisition. Tracking will inevitably be made faster and available in all commercial products. All this will continue the imaging revolution and will provide us with a much better understanding of the structure and pathologies of the vitreo-retinal interface.

Compliance with Ethical Requirements Dr Binder is a consultant for Thrombogenics.

Dr Glittenberg is a consultant for Alcon, Novartis, Thea, Neovista, Oraya, and Zeiss.

The Ludwig Boltzmann Institute received a research grant from Zeiss Meditec.

No animal or human studies were carried out by the authors for this chapter.

References

Binder S, Falkner-Radler CI, Hauger C, Matz H, Glittenberg C (2011) Feasibility of intrasurgical spectral-domain optical coherence tomography. Retina 31(7):1332–1336

Drexler W (2004) Ultrahigh resolution optical coherence tomography. J Biomed Opt 9(1):47–74

Girach A, Kozma-Wiebe P, Pakola S, for the MIVI-TRUST Study Group (2012) Ocriplasmin as treatment for symptomatic vitreomacular adhesion: Phase III trial results. Poster at Knowledge for Growth International Conference, Ghent, Belgium, May 2012

Glittenberg C, Krebs I, Falkner-Radler C, Zeiler F, Haas P, Hagen S, Binder S (2009) Advantages of using a ray-traced, three-dimensional rendering system for spectral domain Cirrus HD-OCT to visualize subtle structures of the vitreoretinal interface. Ophthalmic Surg Lasers Imaging 40(2):127–134

Glittenberg C, Lamar PD, Esmaeelpour M, Zeiler F, Radler CF, Binder S (2012) The use of triamcinolone as a contrast agent for intrasurgical OCT. ARVO Meet Abstr March 26, 53, 2095

Hahn P, Migacz J, O'Connell R, Izatt JA, Toth CA (2013) Unprocessed real-time imaging of vitreoretinal surgical maneuvers using a microscope-integrated spectral-domain optical coherence tomography system. Graefes Arch Clin Exp Ophthalmol 251(1):213–220 [Epub ahead of print]

Krebs I, Glittenberg C, Zeiler F, Binder S (2011) Spectral domain optical coherence tomography for higher precision in the evaluation of vitreoretinal adhesions in exudative age-related macular degeneration. Br J Ophthalmol 95(10):1415–1418, Epub 2011 Jan 26

Mirza RG, Johnson MW, Jampol LM (2007) Optical coherence tomography use in evaluation of the vitreo-retinal interface: a review. Surv Ophthalmol 52(4):397–421

Sebag J (2004) Seeing the invisible: the challenge of imaging vitreous. J Biomed Opt 9(1):38–46

Wojtkowski M, Fercher AF, Leitgeb R (2001) Phase sensitive interferometry in optical coherence tomography. Proc SPIE 4515:250–255

Roy M. Arogyasami and Pravin U. Dugel

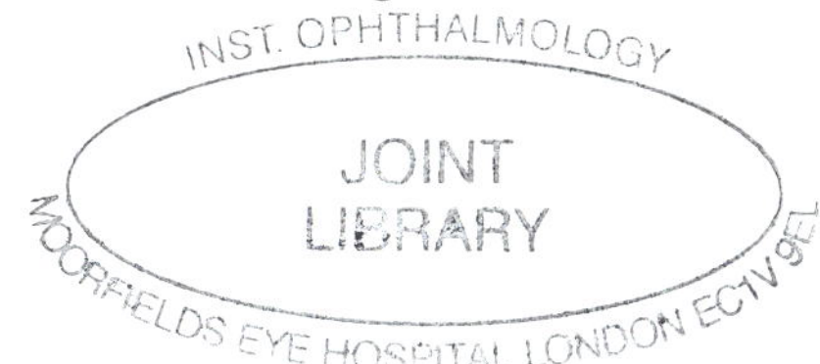

7.1 Macular Hole

7.1.1 Symptoms

Macular holes can cause painless visual loss and distortion which may or may not be progressive. The distorted or decreased vision may go unnoticed as the patient becomes reliant on the other eye. If progression occurs, the hole will likely be noticed as the vision deteriorates. Symptoms of macular holes can greatly vary and do not necessarily reflect changes in funduscopic exam. In a case series of 198 patients with untreated macular hole, only one third of patients had an increase in size of the hole, yet 45 % had decreased visual acuity by at least two lines. When looking at fellow eyes, only 7 % went on to develop a macular hole (Chew et al 1999).

7.1.2 Signs

Macular holes may be noted initially on dilated fundus examination and are easier to detect as they progress. Stage I holes may be difficult to visualize without OCT imaging, particularly when the patient has media opacities. However, stage II, III, and IV holes are easier to diagnose without ancillary studies.

Three clinical tests are frequently used to help diagnose macular holes: the Watzke-Allen test, Amsler Grid, and laser beam aiming test. The Watzke-Allen (W/A) test can be used to confirm suspicion of a macular hole. In this test, the practitioner uses a fundus lens at the slit lamp to aim a thin beam of light on the macula. The beam is moved over the area of macular pathology, and the patient is asked whether they see a break or thinning in the line when the beam of light crosses the macular defect. In a series of 40 patients with macular holes, 39 patients reported the beam of light to be broken or thinned in *either* the horizontal or vertical placement of the light beam (Tanner and Williamson 2000) (Table 7.1).

Although the W/A test, which was originally reported in 1969, may seem antiquated (Watzke and Allen 1969), a recent study compared it with spectral domain OCT in gas-filled eye status post-macular hole repair. At postoperative day 2, only 77.5 % of eyes could yield diagnosable SD OCT images. However, 100 % of the series of 40 patients in the study were able to respond to the W/A test. When obtainable, the accuracy of the SD OCT was significantly better with 31 of 31 patients correctly diagnosed, while only 31 of 40 patients were correctly diagnosed with the W/A test. Thus, the W/A test was still proven useful when used in conjunction with SD OCT (Yamakiri and Sakamoto 2012).

In addition to the W/A test, the laser beam aiming test and Amsler grid are useful in diagnosing patients with macular holes. In a study

R.M. Arogyasami, MD • P.U. Dugel, MD (✉)
Department of Ophthalmology,
Retinal Consultants of Arizona, Phoenix, AZ, USA
e-mail: pdugel@gmail.com

A. Girach, M.D. de Smet (eds.), *Diseases of the Vitreo-Macular Interface*, Essentials in Ophthalmology,
DOI 10.1007/978-3-642-40034-6_7, © Springer-Verlag Berlin Heidelberg 2014

Table 7.1 Watzke-Allen test findings in study

Patient response to W/A test	Number of patients with response
Thinned line with both horizontal and vertical light beam	24
Complete break of line with both horizontal and vertical light beam	9
Thinned in one direction of light beam, broken in the other	6
Line was kinked but not thinned or broken	1

comparing the ability of the three tests to differentiate macular holes versus pseudoholes, the techniques varied in diagnostic capability. The Amsler grid was sensitive but not specific in detection of macular hole; however, the W/A test and to a greater degree the laser beam aiming test were found to be both sensitive and specific (Martinez et al 1994). An image of an Amsler grid with metamorphopsia is shown in Fig. 7.1.

Macular holes vary in size according to stage, but it is also important for the clinician to note signs of posterior vitreous detachment such as a Weiss ring which are seen in stage IV holes. Other tools in the clinic such as ultrasound may be useful in the assessment of macular holes. In a study of 25 eyes, Dugel et al. found that echography was highly correlated with intraoperative characteristics in macular holes for the characteristics of operculum, surrounding subretinal cuff, and complete versus limited posterior vitreous face separation (Dugel et al 1994).

7.1.3 Staging and Prognosis

Staging a macular hole is essential to giving the patient an accurate prognosis. Table 7.2 shows basic guidelines for differentiating the stages, and although this can be done at the slit lamp, ancillary studies such as OCT can confirm findings and be useful in demonstrating pathology to the patient. It is important to recognize and correlate fundus findings with both OCT and fluorescein angiography in order to differentiate macular holes.

The clinical signs of macular holes at stages I, II, III, and IV were elucidated by Gass et al. in the 1970s. Now, we also recognize stage 0 macular

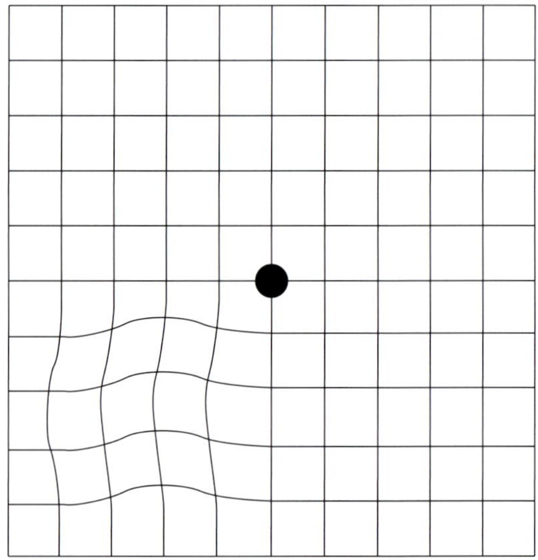

Fig. 7.1 Amsler grid test showing metamorphopsia

holes which are undetectable at the slit lamp but show oblique traction on the fovea at the vitreoretinal interface in OCT images. In a study of 94 patients with macular holes, 24 of the fellow eyes were found to have oblique traction and diagnosed as stage 0 holes. In follow-up of these fellow eyes, 46 % of those with stage 0 holes progressed to full-thickness macular hole, while only 6 % of eyes without stage 0 classification progressed (Chan et al 2004). A more recent classification suggests that the diameter of the hole on OCT is one of the most important prognostic factors in assessing a macular hole. Holes under 250 μm respond well to surgery without any ILM peeling, while it may be required in holes above 400 μm. Pharmacologic release of vitreomacular traction may also be effective in holes under 400 μm (Duker et al. 2013).

7.1.4 Lamellar Holes

Lamellar macular holes are considered aborted macular holes or complications related to chronic cystoid macular edema, high myopia, or other diseases. They can be difficult to differentiate on clinical exam without OCT which shows loss of foveal contour, inner retinal defect, and preserved outer retina and photoreceptors. Lamellar holes are largely found to be stable and do not have

Table 7.2 Macular hole staging

Stage	Full thickness	>400 μM	PVD	Visual acuity	Notable features
0	–	–	–	20/20	Oblique traction of vitreoretinal interface seen on OCT
Ia	–	–	–	20/20–20/40	50 % resolve without intervention
Ib	–	–	–	20/20–20/40	Foveal cyst with cuff of subretinal fluid
II	+	–	–	20/50–20/400	Almost 100 % progression to stage III
III	+	+	–	20/200–20/800	No PVD
IV	+	+	+	20/200–20/800	Weiss ring and complete PVD

progressive loss of visual acuity (Haouchine et al 2004; Witkin et al 2006). Even in high myopes these holes were found to be largely stable. In a case series of 24 eyes with lamellar holes, only 1 eye developed a full-thickness macular hole (Tanaka et al 2011).

7.1.5 Associated Conditions: Trauma, Myopia, etc.

Patient history is an essential component of any clinical evaluation. Although most cases of macular hole are idiopathic, there are some associated conditions such as trauma, myopia, vitrectomy, and family history.

Trauma was the etiology of the first published case of macular holes by Herman Knapp in 1869 (Huang et al 2010). Since then many other associated etiologies have been discovered. In a study comparing idiopathic versus traumatic macular holes, trauma-induced macular holes were noted to be thinner, larger at the base, less circular, and associated with worse visual acuities. Both idiopathic and traumatic holes had a negative correlation between diameter and acuity. Other sources of trauma-related macular holes have been noted in case reports including electrical shock injury (Rajagopal et al. 2010), retinitis sclopetaria (Kunjukunju et al. 2010), and unintentional argon and Nd:YAG laser burns (Bernstein and Steffensmeier 2005; Sou et al. 2003; Lam and Tso 1996).

High myopes are thought to develop macular holes secondary to traction which leads to schisis and ultimately a full-thickness hole (Smiddy et al 2009). Eyes at the atrophic stage in development of choroidal neovascularization have a higher rate of macular hole development and should be periodically monitored with OCT (Shimada et al 2008). In regard to prognosis, patients with myopic macular holes which were not associated with retinal detachment had satisfactory anatomical improvement after vitrectomy. However, the high myopes had poorer visual acuity outcomes in comparison to patients with idiopathic macular hole. Frequently, patients with high myopia and macular hole also develop retinal detachment which is predominantly inferior and bullous in nature (Kumar et al. 2011). Patients with associated retinoschisis around the macular hole in high myopia are thought to do worse post-vitrectomy (Jo et al 2012).

There may be a hereditary component in the development of macular holes. A recent case control study found that 16.7 % of patients with bilateral macular holes had family members with the diagnosis of macular hole. The result was statistically significant even considering confounding variables such as family size and age. This was not necessarily true of patients with unilateral macular hole and may suggest a familial component to the development of bilateral disease (Kay et al. 2012).

Macular holes after vitrectomy are quite rare; in a retrospective chart review only 8 of 3,279 (0.24 %) eyes developed macular holes post-vitrectomy. Both anatomic and functional visual outcome of secondary macular holes was good (Lee et al 2010).

7.1.6 Differential Diagnosis

Many conditions can be confused for macular holes, and these are listed below in Table 7.3 along with differentiating characteristics seen on FA and OCT.

Table 7.3 Differential diagnosis for macular holes with characteristic features on OCT and fluorescein angiography

Diagnosis	OCT	FA
Epiretinal membrane (pseudohole)	Hyperreflective ILM not full-thickness defect	Distortion of fine capillaries in the macula
Cystoid macular edema	Cystoid spaces in the macula	Leakage (not transmission)
Vitreo-macular traction syndrome	Vitreoretinal traction	Variable based on secondary effects
Central areolar pigment epitheliopathy	OCT does not show central full-thickness retinal defects	Transmission/window defect
Pattern dystrophy	Thickened hyperreflective lesion within the RPE	Hypofluorescence in areas of hyperpigmentation
Solar retinopathy/light phototoxicity	Central window defect	RPE hyporeflective with possible hyperreflectivity of the injured neurosensory retina
Choroidal neovascularization	Vascularization, serous PED/RD	Leakage
Central serous chorioretinopathy	Serous PEDs and neurosensory detachments	Pooling in serous PEDs and neurosensory detachments

7.1.7 Clinical Considerations with Repaired Macular Holes

There are numerous considerations in a patient with a repaired macular hole. In the past patients with ICG staining of the internal limiting membrane were found to have retinal pigment epithelial changes that were not consistent with light toxicity. ICG-related retinal damage was later confirmed with multifocal electroretinography studies; triamcinolone membrane blue, and Brilliant Blue were not associated with these issues. The most frequent complications for patients with repaired macular holes are listed in Table 7.4.

7.2 Epiretinal Membrane

7.2.1 Symptoms

An epiretinal membrane (ERM) can range in severity from producing no visual changes to causing extreme metamorphopsia and decreased vision. There are many synonyms for ERMs which refer to the degree of fundus pathology. The term cellophane maculopathy refers to mild disease, and moderate disease is referred to as surface wrinkling retinopathy, premacular gliosis, or fibrosis. In the setting of severe disease,

Table 7.4 Common complications following macular hole surgery

Nuclear sclerosis	60 %
Retinal tears and detachment	10 %
Late reopening	5 %
Light toxicity	Rare
Temporal visual field defects	Possibly secondary to air infusion with drying or ICG toxicity

macular pucker may be chosen as the descriptor for the ERM.

Severe visual loss is uncommon, and in a series of 150 patients with ERMs only four patients had vision below 20/200 with the majority of patients better than 20/50 (Wise 1975). The disease occurs mostly in older populations with over 90 % of cases seen in patients over the age of 50 (Sidd et al. 1982; Charlap et al. 1992).

Rarely, ERMs can cause diplopia if extrafoveal traction occurs. The traction created by the lesion can induce foveal ectopia, and yet visual acuity may not completely deteriorate. Due to disruption of the photoreceptor architecture, patients may also complain of micropsia, macropsia, and metamorphopsia. In a study of 29 eyes, it was found that foveal dystopia was present in 7 eyes and the degree of traction was correlated with worse visual acuity (Lo et al. 2012)

7.2.2 Signs

Epiretinal membranes can be diagnosed at the slit lamp and confirmed with ancillary tests. Thus, it is important to recognize the multitude of associated signs ranging from a mild glistening of the internal limiting membrane found in cellophane maculopathy to distinct gray-white membranes found in macular pucker. In patients with mild ERMs that only have a fine sheen, a red-free filter can aid in visualization. When the ERM is secondary to retinal detachment or severe trauma and inflammation, obvious pigmented and fibrotic areas can be seen.

White areas seen in ERMs are not always due to gliosis – at times the nerve fiber layer will whiten secondary to traction secondary to axoplasmic stasis. This important sign can be discovered at the slit lamp, and documentation can help avoid attempts to peel the nerve fiber layer intraoperatively. If traction in the macula is sufficient, a "tabletop" elevation can show obvious ridges of detachment in the retina. Another key finding is vascular tortuosity and obscuration which lies under the ERM, and many patients have visible retinal striae and distortion of fine macular capillaries leading towards the fovea.

Although the pathogenesis of ERMs is not fully understood, it is likely related to disruptions in the internal limiting membrane (ILM). This may explain why 90 % of eyes with ERMs have posterior vitreous detachment (PVD) which can disrupt the ILM. Yet, some eyes with ERMs do not have a complete PVD but rather show partial perifoveal vitreous detachments on OCT. These partial detachments with epiretinal membranes are not uncommon. In a case series of 207 patients with acute, symptomatic PVDs, 54 patients (26.1 %) had incomplete detachments, and with a mean follow-up of 5 years, 12 of these patients (7.6 %) developed an ERM (Carrero 2012).

ERMs can mimic macular holes by wrinkling the retina around the fovea to create a central circular defect. It can be difficult to distinguish this from a true macular hole; thus, it is referred to as a "macular pseudohole" and will contain retinal tissue in the center of the defect rather than show full-thickness pathology. Up to 8 % of idiopathic ERMs can appear as macular pseudoholes (Sidd et al. 1982).

Unlike true macular holes, pseudoholes do not exhibit yellow RPE deposits in the base of the hole or a surrounding cuff of subretinal fluid. In addition to this, OCT of pseudoholes can demonstrate adjacent retinal wrinkling and hyperreflective ILM. As mentioned in Sect. 8.1, the Watzke-Allen test, laser beam aiming test, and Amsler grid can all be useful in the differentiation of macular holes from ERMs.

7.2.3 Associated Conditions

There are many conditions associated with epiretinal membranes. Some of the most common conditions are listed below:
- Idiopathic
- Diabetes
- Retinal breaks
- Retinal detachment
- Retinal edema
- Retinal vascular occlusions
- Retinitis and choroiditis
- Vitreous hemorrhage
- Vitreous inflammation
- Ophthalmic lasers and surgery
- Cryopexy
- Blunt or penetrating ocular trauma

7.2.4 Staging and Prognosis

There is no official staging for epiretinal membranes. However, as mentioned previously, terms such as cellophane maculopathy imply mild pathology and macular pucker refer to more severe cases. In regard to prognosis, a study of 324 patients found that at 33 months follow-up, 49.5 % maintained visual acuity within one line of initial acuity, 13.1 % were greater than one line better, and 37.4 % were beyond one line worse. Although rare, spontaneous separation of the membrane with improvement in visual acuity and decreased symptoms has been reported (Messner 1977).

7.2.5 Differential Diagnosis

Epiretinal membranes are extremely common occurring in 5 % of all patients and up to 20 % of those over 70 (Clarkson and Green 1977). Frequent conditions that can be confused for ERMs include macular hole, tractional retinal detachment, and macular edema.

7.3 Vitreo-macular Traction Syndrome and Related Conditions

7.3.1 Symptoms

Vitreo-macular traction syndrome (VMTS) can induce a variety of pathological conditions in the eye and may present with decreased visual acuity, metamorphopsia, micropsia, macropsia, and photopsias. Symptoms are frequently mild, but some patients present with vision worse than 20/50 and progressive visual loss. These patients are likely suffering from traction-induced cystoid macular edema or other pathologies.

7.3.2 Signs

Vitreo-macular traction syndrome is now considered a spectrum of disorders which induce secondary pathology. These conditions include macular holes, cystoid macular edema, epiretinal membranes, and retinoschisis; the signs associated with these are covered at length in this and other chapters. Vitreo-macular adhesion can also be associated with macular degeneration. Due to these secondary conditions, VMTS is difficult to diagnose with specificity based on clinical exam alone, but in conjunction with OCT, the task is made easier. Absence of a Weiss ring can be useful in ruling out stage IV macular holes, and earlier stages can be easily confused for VMTS. The images below show the nature of the vitreous in complete posterior vitreous detachment versus vitreo-macular traction syndrome (Figs. 7.2, 7.3, 7.4, 7.5).

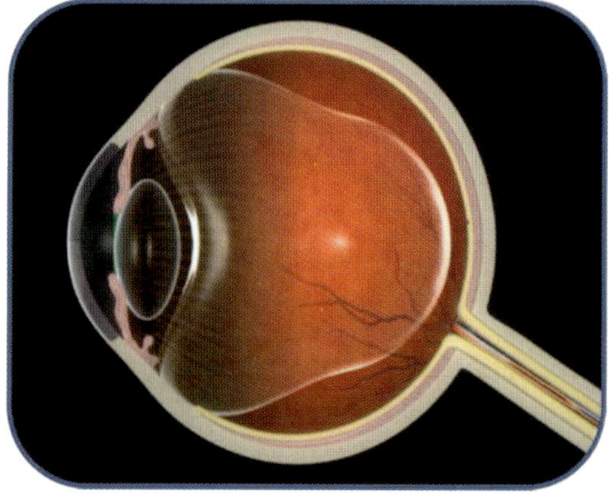

Fig. 7.2 Complete PVD

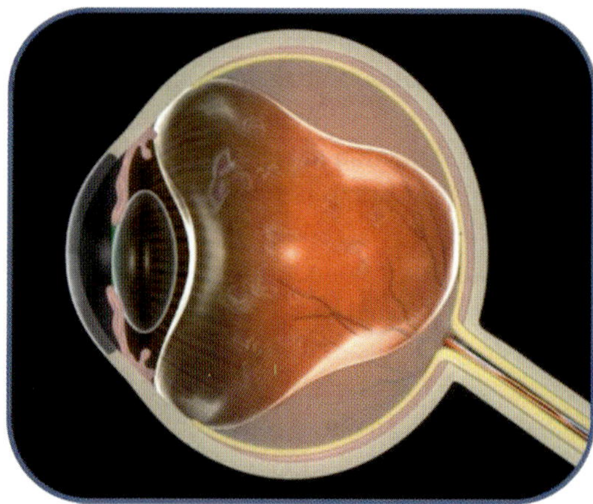

Fig. 7.3 Vitreo-macular adhesion/traction

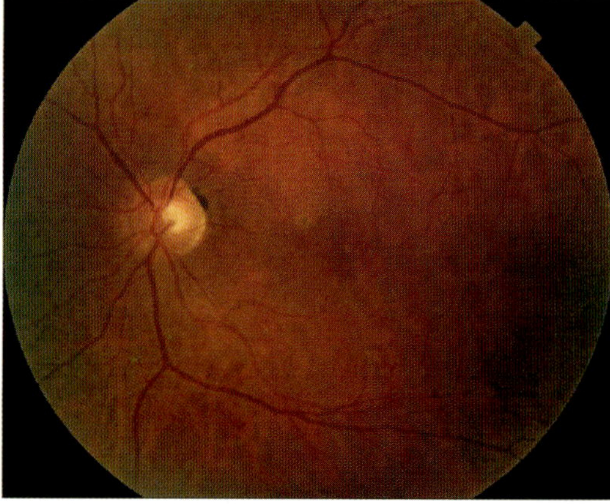

Fig. 7.4 Fundus photo of vitreo-macular traction in the fovea

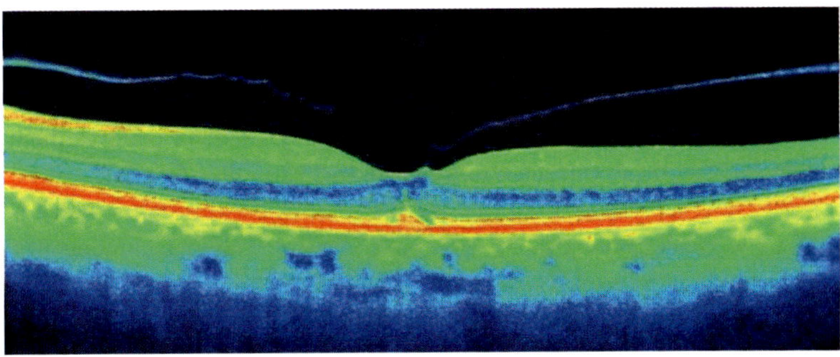

Fig. 7.5 OCT of vitreo-macular traction in the fovea

7.3.3 Vitreofoveal Traction Syndrome

It is not clear whether vitreofoveal traction syndrome (VFTS) is a separate entity from VMTS or part of the spectrum of macular holes. It is characterized by a more focal vitreous attachment that can vary in degrees of traction. The patient may exhibit the signs and symptoms associated with VMTS. The clinical course may be stable, progressive, or have spontaneous resolution.

7.3.4 Myopic Traction Maculopathy

High myopia has been noted to have tractional effects at the vitreoretinal interface and is referred to as myopic traction maculopathy (MTM). A multitude of findings are seen in MTM with retinoschisis being the most common. Other associations include macular hole, epiretinal membrane, and macular edema which are further discussed in their corresponding sections of Chap. 8.

Retinoschisis affects over half of eyes with myopic traction. In 2004, Panozzo et al. studied 125 eyes of patients with high myopia. These patients had an average spherical equivalent of −16.93 diopters, and epiretinal traction was found in 46.4 % with retinal damage in 34.4 %. In other studies, Benhamou et al. (2002) showed that retinoschisis can affect the inner or outer layers of the fovea and noted that cystoid spaces may occur. They concluded that most patients have stable visual acuity with tractional retinoschisis unless they developed a macular hole.

Findings associated with myopic traction maculopathy:

- Retinoschisis
- Shallow retinal detachment
- Macular edema
- Epiretinal membrane
- Macular hole
- Retinal microfolds

Fujimoto et al. reviewed 21 patients with high myopia and retinoschisis. They found that ILM detachments in the superior or inferior peripheral macula are associated with foveal retinal detachments. The researchers concluded that strong tractional forces on the ILM are likely transmitted beyond the schisis to the outer retina and produce retinal detachments of the fovea (Fujimoto et al 2010). Retinal microfolds are another key finding in high myopia which are likely secondary to the inflexibility of retinal vessels in an elongated eye. Retinal microfolds are not uncommon, having a prevalence of 2.9 % in highly myopic eyes (Sayanagi et al. 2005).

7.3.5 Diabetic Traction Maculopathy

Diabetes has classically been thought to cause edema by breakdown of the blood retinal barrier, but new evidence shows that in select cases traction may be a contributing factor. Traction-related macular edema is noted to be diffused rather than cystoid. Karatas et al. showed that diffuse macular edema that was not responsive to laser is frequently associated with vitreopapillary traction (Karatas et al. 2005). Bandello et al.

(2003) suggested a new system of classification be employed to describe the various etiologies of diabetic macular edema: taut posterior hyaloid, retinovascular dysfunction, and traction. They suggested that these various etiologies be further investigated, so that tailoring treatment regimens may have greater efficacy.

In a study of 87 eyes, Haller et al. showed that macular edema in diabetes that was associated with vitreo-macular traction was highly responsive to vitrectomy. Many eyes in the study had additional intraoperative treatments including epiretinal membrane peel, internal limiting membrane peel, steroid injections, and panretinal photocoagulation. Patient outcomes showed that 28–49 % of patients had improved visual outcomes and 13–33 % had a decrease in vision. In these procedures, there was no increase in intraoperative complications.

Vitrectomy may be beneficial in diabetics with macular edema regardless of whether traction is present. Aboutable and Kalvodova (2005) found that surgery on eyes both with and without vitreo-macular traction resulted in positive outcomes and noted that a shorter duration of macular edema portends a favorable prognosis. In support of this idea, a pathologic analysis performed by Gandorfer et al. (2005) on 61 vitrectomized eyes showed that in diffuse diabetic macular edema, the vitreo-macular interface had a layer of native vitreous collagen with variable cell types. However, resolution of edema was not dependent on the presence and removal of contractile membranes. In eyes without any traction, removal of epimacular tissue also led to fluid resorption.

Traditionally traction on the retina from diabetes causes both retinal breaks and retinal detachments which can be long-standing and develop in the macula. Extramacular detachments are observed and can be stable. However, these retinal detachments and breaks can have classic symptoms of flashes, floaters, and decreased vision.

7.3.6 Differential Diagnosis

Vitreo-macular and other traction syndromes can induce secondary disorders such as macular holes, cystoid macular edema, epiretinal membranes, and retinoschisis. Often without OCT imaging the primary diagnosis is not correctly noted as a tractional syndrome. Less commonly, the diagnosis is mistaken for central serous chorioretinopathy, RPE tears, and tractional retinal detachments in the macula.

Conclusion

In conclusion, vitreo-macular interface disease has multiple presentations that can produce significant visual disturbances. These conditions include macular holes, epiretinal membranes, and vitreo-macular traction with resultant retinal schisis or edema. Slit lamp examination with a macular lens is essential for proper diagnosis and initiating further workup. Beyond this, using the Watzke-Allen test, laser beam aiming test, and Amsler grid can be useful before any imaging technology is used. Optical coherence tomography, fluorescein angiography, and fundus photos are important for confirming, prognosticating, and documenting the diagnosis. It is important to recognize that vitreo-macular disease can be related to many forms of ocular and systemic pathology such as diabetes, myopia, and uveitis, which may need further workup. Thus, vitreo-macular interface diseases are an important part of any ophthalmologist's differential diagnosis and should be well understood.

Compliance with Ethical Requirements Dr Roy Arogyasami declares that he has no conflict of interests.

Dr Dugel has or is a consultant for Abbott, Acucela, Acuity, Alcon, Alimera, Allergan, ANI Research, Arizona Research Center, Bausch & Lomb, Bayer, Carl T Hayden Medical Research Foundation, CoMentis, Control Delivery Systems, Dedicated Clinical Research, Dedicated Phase 1, DRCR Network, Lilly, Eyetech, Fovea, Geneara, Genentech, Genzyme, GSK, Immusol, iScience, JAEB, Johns Hopkins Research, JDRF, Lpath, Lux Bio, Macusight, Merck, NEI/NIH, Neovista, Novartis, Novagali, Occulogix, Oculex, Ophthotech, Opko, Optimedica, Othera, Ovation, Pfizer, Quark, Regeneron, Santen, Southwest Kidney Institute, SurModics, ThromboGenics, TopCon, Univ of California, and VitreoRetinal Technologies.

No animal or human studies were carried out by the authors for this chapter.

References

Aboutable T, Kalvodova B (2005) Vitrectomy for diabetic cystoid macular edema – results of 72 cases. Klin Monbl Augenheilkd 222(8):643–8, In German

Bandello F, Pognuz R, Polito A, Pirracchio A, Menchini F, Ambesi M (2003) Diabetic macular edema: classification, medical and laser therapy. Semin Ophthalmol 18(4):251–258

Benhamou N, Massin P, Haouchine B, Erginay A, Gaudric A (2002) Macular retinoschisis in highly myopic eyes. Am J Ophthalmol 133(6):794–800

Bernstein PS, Steffensmeier A (2005) Optical coherence tomography before and after repair of a macular hole induced by an unintentional argon laser burn. Arch Ophthalmol 123(3):404–405

Carrero JL (2012) Incomplete posterior vitreous detachment: prevalence and clinical relevance. Am J Ophthalmol 153(3):497–503, Epub 2011 Nov 8

Chan A, Duker JS, Schuman JS, Fujimoto JG (2004) Stage 0 macular holes: observations by optical coherence tomography. Ophthalmology 111(11):2027–2032

Charlap RS, Yagoda AD, Debbi S, Bodine SR, Walsh JB, Henkind P (1992) Idiopathic preretinal macular gliosis: a retrospective study of 200 patients. Ann Ophthalmol 24(10):381–385

Chew EY, Sperduto RD, Hiller R, Nowroozi L, Seigel D, Yanuzzi LA, Burton TC, Seddon JM, Gragoudas ES, Haller JA, Blair NP, Farber M (1999) Clinical course of macular holes: The Eye Disease Case–control study. Arch Ophthalmol 117(2):242–246

Clarkson JG, Green WR, Massof D (1977) A histopathologic review of 168 cases of preretinal membrane. Am J Ophthalmol 84:1

Duker JS, Kaiser PK, Binder S, de Smet MD, Gaudric A, Reichel E, Sadda SR, Sebag J, Spaide RF, Stalmans P (2013) The international vitreomacular traction study group classification of vitreomacular adhesion, traction, and macular hole. Ophthalmology 120(12):2611–9

Dugel PU, Smiddy WE, Byrne SF, Hughes JR, Gass JD (1994) Macular hole syndromes: echographic findings with clinical correlation. Ophthalmology 101(5):815–821

Fujimoto M, Hangai M, Suda K, Yoshimura N (2010) Features associated with foveal retinal detachment in myopic macular retinoschisis. Am J Ophthalmol 150(6):863–870, Epub 2010 Oct 16

Gandorfer A, Rohleder M, Grosselfinger S, Haritoglou C, Ulbig M, Kampik A (2005) Epiretinal pathology of diffuse diabetic macular edema associated with vitreomacular traction. Am J Ophthalmol 139(4):638–652

Haouchine B, Massin P, Tadayoni R, Erginay A, Gaudric A (2004) Diagnosis of macular pseudoholes and lamellar macular holes by optical coherence tomography. Am J Ophthalmol 138:732–739

Huang J, Liu X, Wu Z, Sadda S (2010) Comparison of full-thickness traumatic macular holes and idiopathic macular holes by optical coherence tomography. Graefes Arch Clin Exp Ophthalmol 248(8):1071–1075, Epub 2010 Feb 24

Jo Y, Ikuno Y, Nishida K (2012) Retinoschisis: a predictive factor in vitrectomy for macular holes without retinal detachment in highly myopic eyes. Br J Ophthalmol 96(2):197–200, Epub 2011 May 17

Karatas M, Ramirez JA, Ophir A (2005) Diabetic vitreopapillary traction and macular oedema. Eye 19:676–682. doi:10.1038/sj.eye.6701622, Published online 3 September 2004

Kay CN, Pavan PR, Small LB, Zhang T, Zamba GK, Cohen SM (2012) Familial trends in a population with macular holes. Retina 32(4):754–759

Knapp H (1869) Ueber isolirte zerreissungen der aderhaut in folge von traumen auf dem augapfel. Arch Augenheilkd 1:6–29

Kumar A, Tinwala S, Gogia V, Sinha S.(2012) Clinical presentation and surgical outcomes in primary myopic macular hole retinal detachment. Eur J Ophthalmol. 2012;22(3):450–455

Kunjukunju N, Navarro A, Oliver S, Olson J, Patel C, Garcia G, Mandava N, Quiroz-Mercado H (2010) Bilateral macular hole formation secondary to sclopetaria caused by shockwaves transmitted by a posterior vector: case report. BMC Ophthalmol 10:6

Lam TT, Tso MO (1996) Retinal injury by neodymium: YAG laser. Retina 16(1):42–46

Lee SH, Park KH, Kim JH, Heo JW, Yu HG, Yu YS, Chung H (2010) Secondary macular hole formation after vitrectomy. Retina 30(7):1072–1077

Lo D, Heussen F, Ho HK, Narala R, Gasperini J, Bertoni B, Na M, Walsh AC, Fawzi AA (2012) Structural and functional implications of severe foveal dystopia in epiretinal membranes. Retina 32(2):340–348

Martinez J, Smiddy WE, Kim J, Gass JD (1994) Differentiating macular holes from macular pseudoholes. Am J Ophthalmol 117(6):762–767

Messner KH (1977) Spontaneous separation of preretinal macular fibrosis. Am J Ophthalmol 83(9):1977

Rajagopal J, Shetty SB, Kamath AG, Kamath GG (2010) Macular hole following electrical shock injury. Can J Ophthalmol 45(2):187–188

Sayanagi K, Ikuno Y, Gomi F, Tano Y (2005) Retinal vascular microfolds in highly myopic eyes. Am J Ophthalmol 139(4):658–663

Shimada N, Ohno-Matsui K, Yoshida T, Futagami S, Tokoro T, Mochizuki M (2008) Development of macular hole and macular retinoschisis in eyes with myopic choroidal neovascularization. Am J Ophthalmol 145(1):155–161, Epub 2007 Nov 7

Sidd RJ, Fine SL, Owens SL, Patz A (1982) Idiopathic preretinal gliosis. Am J Ophthalmol 94(1):44–48

Smiddy WE, Kim SS, Lujan BJ, Gregori G (2009) Myopic traction maculopathy: spectral domain optical coherence tomographic imaging and a hypothesized mechanism. Ophthalmic Surg Lasers Imaging 40(2):169–173

Sou R, Kusaka S, Ohji M, Gomi F, Ikuno Y, Tano Y (2003) Optical coherence tomographic evaluation of a surgically treated traumatic macular hole secondary to Nd:YAG laser injury. Am J Ophthalmol 135(4):537–539

Tanaka Y, Shimada N, Moriyama M, Hayashi K, Yoshida T, Tokoro T, Ohno-Matsui K (2011) Natural history of lamellar macular holes in highly myopic eyes. Am J Ophthalmol 152(1):96–99.e1, Epub 2011 May 12

Tanner V, Williamson TH (2000) Watzke-Allen slit beam test in macular holes confirmed by optical coherence tomography. Arch Ophthalmol 118(8):1059–1063

Watzke RC, Allen L (1969) Subjective slitbeam sign for macular disease. Am J Ophthalmol 68(3): 449–453

Wise GN (1975) Clinical features of idiopathic preretinal macular fibrosi. Schoenberg lecture. Am J Ophthalmol 79(3):349–357

Witkin AJ, Ko TH, Fujimoto JG et al (2006) Redefining lamellar holes and the vitreomacular interface: an ultrahigh-resolution optical coherence tomography study. Ophthalmology 113:388–397

Yamakiri K, Sakamoto T (2012) Early diagnosis of macular hole closure of a gas-filled eye with Watzke-Allen slit beam test and spectral domain optical coherence tomography. Retina 32(4):767–772

Vitreo-macular Traction and Age-Related Macular Degeneration

Susanne Binder and Ilse Krebs

8.1 Background

As age-related macular degeneration is considered a multifactorial disease with its origin in the choroid, the vitreous in this disease group was of little interest for a long time. However prior studies using ultrasound (US) examinations found a higher incidence of attached posterior hyaloid in AMD patients as usually expected in this age group, but no differentiation between wet and dry or active and inactive disease was performed (Ondez and Yilmaz 2000; Weber Krause and Eckardt 1997).

When submacular surgery became popular after Mathew Thomas' reports of successful subfoveal membrane removal in patients with neovascularisation related to histoplasmosis (Thomas 1991), many vitreoretinal surgeons started to remove neovascular complexes also in AMD patients. While visual results with this approach were disappointing and improved methods have been used – like RPE transplantation in suspensions as well as in sheets – what most of us had observed was that during surgery the posterior

S. Binder, MD (✉) • I. Krebs, MD
Department of Ophthalmology,
Rudolf Foundation Clinic,
Teaching Hospital of the Medical University of Vienna,
Juchgasse 25, A 1030 Vienna, Austria

Ludwig Boltzmann Institute for Retinology
and Biomicroscopic Laser Surgery,
Rudolf Foundation Clinic, Juchgasse 25,
A 1030, Vienna, Austria
e-mail: susanne.binder@wienkav.at

hyaloid was found much more often attached than detached. Rather surprising in this elderly group of patients. in our own cases of submacular surgery for NV, we described an attached posterior hyaloid in 83 % in 2004 (Binder et al. 2004).

In addition, we frequently observed a central vitreo-macular adhesion surrounded by a shallow vitreous detachment in eyes treated with photodynamic therapy by stratus OCT. Several other colleagues have made similar observations (Devin 2003), so we decided to look for some proof.

8.1.1 AMD-Vitreous Studies

The first study was a prospective comparative study where we included patients with exudative AMD, dry AMD and age-matched controls. To guarantee that a complete posterior hyaloid detachment would not be overlooked, US examinations were performed in addition to OCTs. As OCT has only a vertical depth of several millimetres, at the time the study was initiated, only dense vitreous membranes in front of the retina could be visualised with OCT. On the retina it was and is still not possible to determine whether the vitreous is completely adherent or completely detached. 163 eyes of 163 patients were included in this study. With US examination we could show that a complete posterior detachment was present in 71.9 % of eyes with dry AMD and in 60.7 % of age-matched controls, but in patients with wet AMD, only 34 % had a detached posterior hyaloid (p-0.0002, p-0.014). Vice versa a partial PVD in

A. Girach, M.D. de Smet (eds.), *Diseases of the Vitreo-Macular Interface*, Essentials in Ophthalmology,
DOI 10.1007/978-3-642-40034-6_8, © Springer-Verlag Berlin Heidelberg 2014

the periphery with a centrally attached posterior hyaloid was detected in 30.0 % of eyes with exudative AMD, but only in 12.3 % of eyes with non-exudative AMD and 5.4 % of controls (p-0.02, p-0.003). Using OCT a persistent adhesion in the central macula surrounded by a detached vitreous cortex was detected in more than a third (36 %) of eyes with exudative AMD, but only in 7 % in eyes with dry AMD and 10.7 % in the control eyes ($p<0.0001$,p-0.002) (Krebs et al. 2007). As we wanted to exclude the influence of genetic and environmental factors, the following prospective studies included only patients with wet AMD in one eye and dry AMD in the partner eye. Simultaneously we divided also cases with active and advanced AMD. These studies were conducted in collaboration with Jerry Sebag, chair of the VRM Institute, Huntington Beach, and Lawrence Yanuzzi's Group in New York. 78 eyes of 39 patients were included; in 29 patients, the AMD was active and in 10 patients an inactive,

terminal AMD was present. By US examination a complete PVD was detected in 69 % of eyes with dry AMD compared to only 21 % in wet AMD (p-0.002). With OCT a vitreo-macular adhesion was found in 38 % in wet AMD eyes, while only 10 % had a vitreo-macular adhesion in the dry cases (p-0008). However, when we looked at the comparison between active and inactive forms of AMD, these differences were no longer detectable; only 2 cases out of 10 showed vitreo-macular adhesion on the fovea in eyes with disciform scars and none had a vitreo-macular adhesion in eyes with geographic atrophy (p-0.48). These results did support our earlier findings in active cases of AMD but showed that in end-stage AMD this difference is no longer significant. Obviously the vitreous separates at very late age when end-stage AMD is reached (Robison et al. 2009). Unfortunately the vitreous does not separate during intravitreal application of anti-VEGF, what is demonstrated in the picture below (Fig. 8.1).

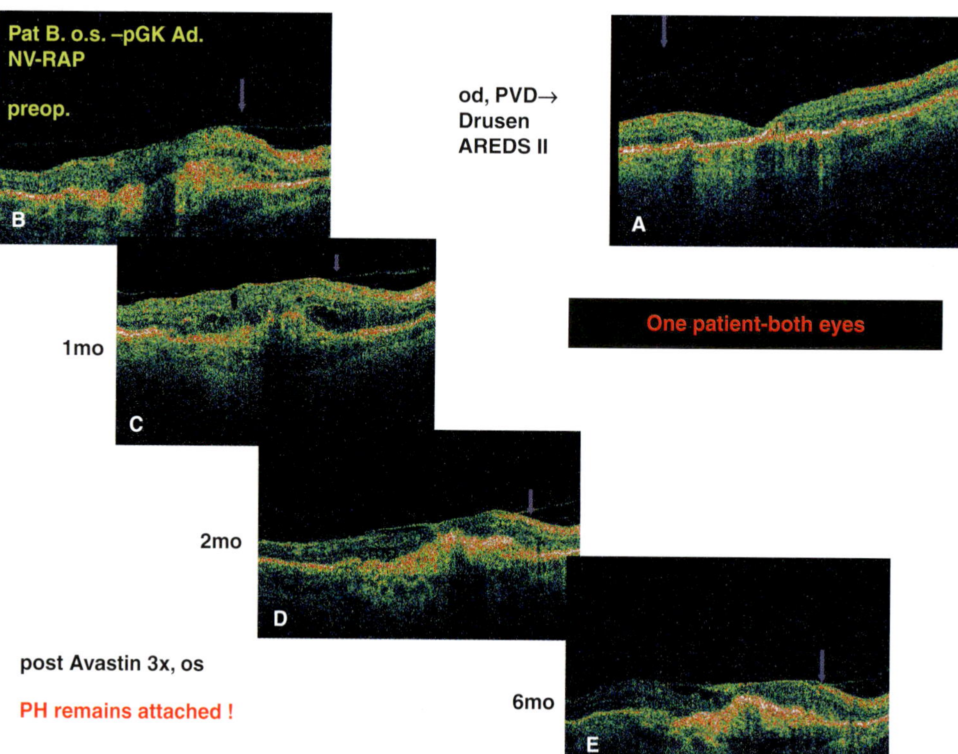

Fig. 8.1 OCT – a patient with wet, neovascular AMD in his left eye, where the vitreous is adherent over the lesion and shows a shallow vitreous detachment at both sides (pic A *left superior*). Pic B *right superior*: right partner eye of the same patient with a detached posterior hyaloid and dry AMD consisting of drusen (AREDS 2). Pic C, D, E *left*: sequence of OCT pictures after anti-VEGF treatment shows still vitreo-macular adhesion

During our studies, we observed that traction is different over these membranes, the most important information about traction height and forces we did receive from Carl Glittenberg's 3D visualisations of the HD OCT pictures. For example, when we cut the 3D complex exactly in the area with the highest vitreous traction, we detected that this was the location where the NV took its origin (Fig. 8.2).

To prove our hypothesis, we studied eyes with vitreo-macular adhesion/traction in a series of 30 eyes and used 2 different available HD OCT (Cirrus/Zeiss Meditec and Spectralis) and performed 3D visualisation (see Chap. 6).

We could show that the area of adhesion corresponded in 100 % with the localisation of the CNV. Interestingly there was a high proportion of retinal angiomatous proliferation (RAP) lesions in this group (50 %); 46 % were occult lesions and 3.3 % had classic lesions. In more than half of cases (56 %), there were extrafoveal adhesions and also the CNVs were juxtafoveal (Fig. 8.3a, b). In 83 % vitreopapillary traction was observed in addition.

When these cases were followed for 12 months, 76.7 % of VMT/adhesion remained unchanged, 10 % developed a posterior vitreous detachment (PVD) and in 13.3 % the traction increased or adhesions did converse to traction (Krebs et al. 2011).

The high incidence of vitreopapillary traction in these eyes is certainly interesting and very often also observed in macular hole (MH) cases. Usually the macular adhesion seems to separate before the papillary adhesion separates. Surgically the papillary adhesion (Weiss ring) is often hard to separate. Strong arrow formed tractions develop in these cases between optic disc and macula, and we believe that it clearly enhances NV growth or MH enlargement (Fig. 8.4).

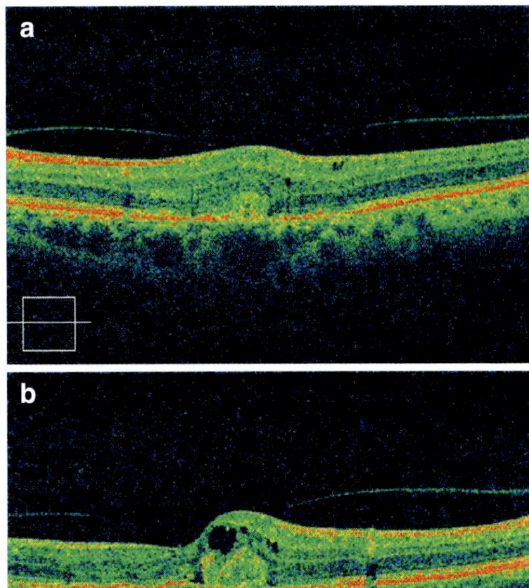

Fig. 8.3 (**a**) Vitreo-macular adhesion – extrafoveal. (**b**) Development of Rap 2 lesion also extrafoveal

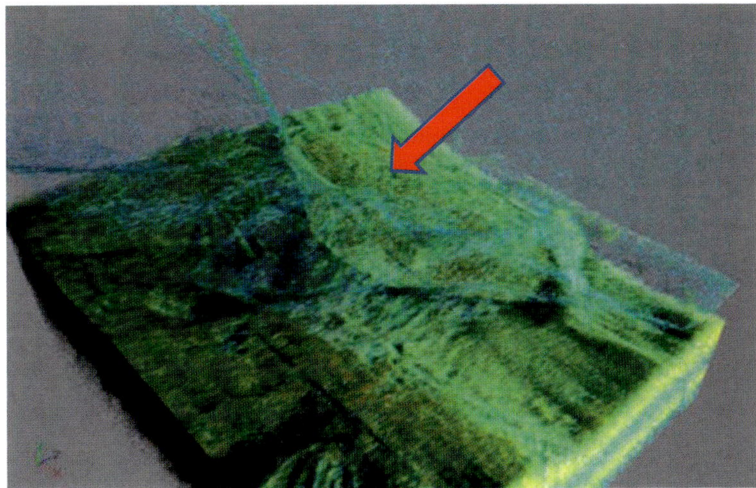

Fig. 8.2 3D HD OCT of vitreo-macular traction in AMD patient. Area of highest traction (*arrow*) is in the location of the NV origin

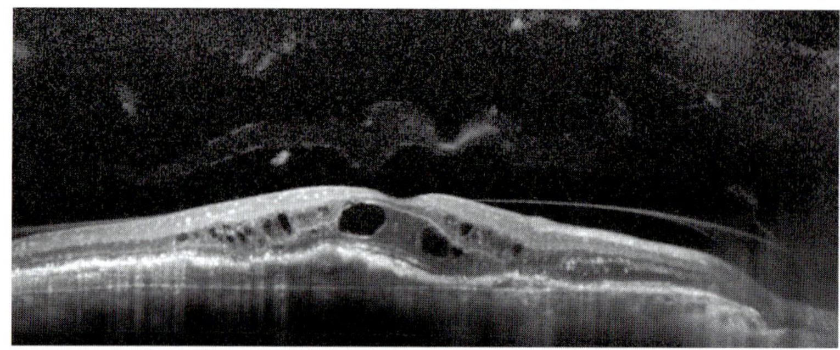

Fig. 8.4 HD OCT of a case with NV AMD where vitreous is separated between optic disc and the fovea, creating an eccentric nasal traction on the macular area

8.2 Pathogenesis

Now, what is the pathogenesis of this abnormal vitreo-macular adhesion we found in exudative AMD? There are at least three possible ways which might all be present with different gravity at the same time:

Nr 1 is the presence of a chronic, low-grade inflammation in the macular region during disease development which induces adhesion in the foveal area (Anderson and Mullins 2002).

Nr 2 is based on the theory that an attached vitreous prevents normal diffusion of oxygen and nutrients required by the metabolically active cells of the macula, thus triggering neovascularisation (Holz 2004).

Nr 3 might be the fact that an attached posterior vitreous confines pro-angiogenetic cytokines in the macula and contributes to the development of neovascularisation (Adamis and Shima 2005).

At this point it is important to mention that AMD is certainly a multifactorial disease, and our findings about the abnormal behaviour of the vitreous can only contribute but do not exclude other factors of disease origin.

Whether an attached hyaloid prevents efficacy of anti-VEGF treatment and is more frequent in nonresponders is examined in current studies. Before numbers of nonresponders are given, a clear definition must be given. In several reports it was agreed that a "nonresponder" to anti-VEGF therapy is a case where there is vision loss of more than three lines, no reduction of central retinal thickness (CRT) on OCT and an increase of lesion size observed on fluorescein angiography (FA). In a retrospective evaluation of 334 eyes treated with either bevacizumab (Avastin*) or ranibizumab (Lucentis*) overall 13.5 % of cases were "nonresponders" with no difference between the drug used. Interestingly when we looked at the presence or absence of vitreo-macular traction/adhesion in these cases, 40.7 % of nonresponders had VM adhesion/traction, while only 8.4 % of eyes responding to therapy had a VM adhesion, again a significant difference.

One would speculate that vitreous separation in these cases, either enzymatically or surgically, might improve treatment effect in exudative AMD with adherent posterior vitreous.

8.3 The Egg or the Hen?

Finally, one would be certainly interested to find out how the evolution of these processes is. Does vitreous adhesion/traction cause neovascularisation in AMD or does the evolving NV process inhibit the vitreous from separation? In short, is the risk of neovascular AMD connected with posterior hyaloid adhesion? When we looked at partner eyes in our wet AMD studies, we found a significant correlation between the risk (AREDS) to develop CNV in dry AMD and attached PH (odds ratio=0.065, 95 % CI for odds ratio=[0.012, 0.362], p-value=0.00178). After 2 years, 6 of 56 eyes developed CNV, 5 of these eyes had an attached posterior vitreous, but the numbers were small. Therefore, we are conducting a prospective study where we look at the posterior hyaloid behaviour using US, OCT and autofluorescence in 6 months interval in patients with dry AMD(AREDS 2 and 3) over 2 years.

Conclusion

We have shown in several studies that VM adhesion plays an important role in AMD and might actually be also an additional risk factor for the development of NV AMD. Traction forces do play a role in the location and origin of NV. As AMD is most likely induced by choroidal ischaemia creating low-grade inflammation and leading to confinement of pro-angiogenetic cytokines in NV AMD, additional hypoxia coming from an attached vitreous could definitely aggravate the disease process. The fact that nonresponders to anti-VEGF treatment did show a sign, higher incidence of vitreo-macular adhesion underlined this. As intravitreal treatments with anti-VEGF do not accelerate or support vitreous separation, enzymatic vitreous separation could clearly enhance the prognosis in this patients with wet AMD and persistent vitreo-macular adhesion or traction.

Compliance with Ethical Requirements Dr Binder is a consultant for ThromboGenics. Dr Krebs declares that she has no conflicts of interest. The Ludwig Boltzmann Institute received a research grant from Zeiss Meditec. No animal or human studies were carried out by the authors for this chapter.

References

Adamis AP, Shima D (2005) The role of vascular endothelial growth factor in ocular health and disease. Retina 25(2):111–118

Anderson DH, Mullins RF (2002) A role for local inflammation in the formation of drusen in the aging eye. Am J Ophthalmol 134(3):411–431

Binder S, Krebs I, Hilgers R et al (2004) Outcome of transplantation of autologous retinal pigment epithelium in age-related macular degeneration. A prospective trial. Invest Ophthalmol Vis Sci 45:4151–4160

Douvin F (2003) Oral communication. 5th St Christophs vitrectomy course. Wengen

Holz FG (2004) Pathogenesis of lesions in late age-related macular disease. Am J Ophthalmol 137(3):504–510

Krebs I, Brannath W, Glittenberg C, Zeiler F, Sebag J, Binder S (2007) Posterior vitreomacular adhesion: a potential risk factor for exudative age-related macular degeneration? Am J Ophthalmol 144(5):741–746

Krebs I, Glittenberg G, Binder S et al (2011) Spectral domain optical coherence tomography for higher precision in the evaluation of vitreoretinal adhesions in exudative age-related macular degeneration. Br J Ophthalmol 95(10):1415–1418

Ondez F, Yilmaz G, Acar MA et al (2000) Role of the vitreous in age-related macular degeneration. Jpn J Ophthalmol 44(1):91–93

Robison CD, Krebs I, Binder S, Barbazetto IA, Kotsolis AI, Yannuzzi LA, Sadun AA, Sebag J (2009) Vitreomacular adhesion in active and end-stage age-related macular degeneration. Am J Ophthalmol 148(1):79–82

Thomas MA (1991) Surgical removal of subretinal neovascularisation in the presumed ocular histoplasmosis syndrome. Am J Ophthalmol 111:1–7

Weber Krause B, Eckardt C (1997) Incidence of posterior vitreous detachment in the elderly. Ophthalmologe 94:619–623

Treatment Paradigm for Vitreo-macular Interface Diseases

9

Matteo Cereda

9.1 Treatment Paradigm for VMI Diseases

When Machemer introduced vitrectomy, it heralded a revolution in ophthalmic care (Machemer et al. 1971). Ophthalmologists were now able to enter the posterior pole and manage it from the inside by surgery. Similarly shocking was the introduction of retinotomy by Zivojnovic. To cut the retina was no more a heresy and could be also a necessity (Zivojnovic and Claes 1990). In the 1980s, removal of epimacular proliferations became routine, and in 1990, Morris et al. reported the first cases of intentional internal limiting membrane removal (Morris et al. 1990). Vitreoretinal surgeons have progressively been able to treat pathologies of the posterior pole. In the last two decades, improvement in surgical techniques and the development of finer surgical tools has allowed ophthalmologists to deal with a wide series of macular disorders. Here we present the paradigm of surgery, based on literature and on experience, of the most frequent vitreo-macular interface diseases.

M. Cereda, MD
Department of Biomedical and Clinical Science
"Luigi Sacco", Eye Clinic, Sacco Hospital,
University of Milan, Milano, Italy
e-mail: matteo.cereda@gmail.com

9.2 Epiretinal Membranes

Epiretinal membrane (ERM) was first described in 1865 (Iwanoff 1865) as an avascular, fibrocellular membrane that proliferates on the inner surface of the ILM. They are composed of different proportions of glial cells, RPE cells, macrophages, fibrocytes, myofibroblasts and collagen fibres (Kampik et al. 1980; Trese et al. 1983). Most ERMs are visually benign and do not require surgery. Still, ERM contraction can cause morphologic distortions of the retinal surface and lead to functional changes such as metamorphopsia and decreased visual acuity. In most eyes, however, once a membrane has been present for several months, further decline of visual acuity is uncommon (Gass 1987). If vision worsens, other ocular conditions such as cataract or retinal pathologies should be suspected. Vitreoretinal surgery is performed when an ERM that has caused significant visual loss. The indication for surgery from one patient to the other, but surgery usually is reserved for those cases in which progressive vision impairment is documented over time. Surgery should also be considered if the patient suffers debilitating metamorphopsia and requires better vision for his daily activities.

The goal of treatment is to remove the ERM and release the retinal distortion. Although some ERMs may resolve spontaneously (Meyer et al. 2004), most require surgical removal. Given that the ILM may act as a scaffold for cell proliferation (Hisatomi et al. 2005), peeling of the ILM may

A. Girach, M.D. de Smet (eds.), *Diseases of the Vitreo-Macular Interface*, Essentials in Ophthalmology,
DOI 10.1007/978-3-642-40034-6_9, © Springer-Verlag Berlin Heidelberg 2014

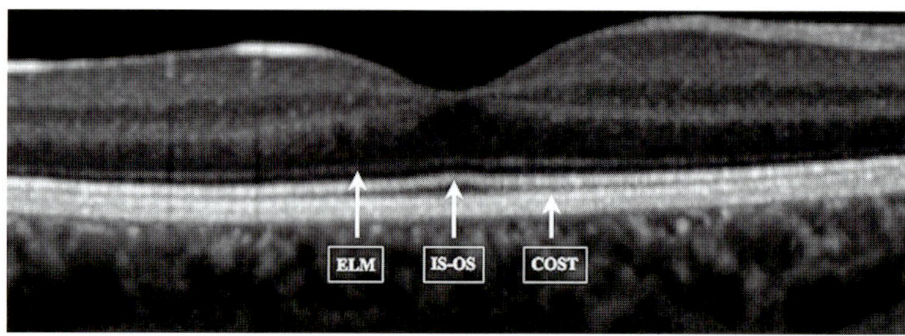

Fig. 9.1 Outer retinal layers on SD-OCT. Outer retinal layers as defined on SD-OCT in a normal retina. *ELM* external limiting membrane, *IS-OS* inner-segment, outer-segment junction of photoreceptors, *COST* cone outer segment tips

ensure the complete removal of the ERM but also decrease the rate of recurrence (Park et al. 2003). Recurrence of the ERM, when ERM and ILM peeling are combined, has been observed in less than 9 % of cases (Bovey et al. 2004). This rate of recurrence is higher, between 7.5 and 56 %, after surgical removal of the ERM alone (Grewing and Mester 1996; Kwok et al. 2005 and Park et al. 2003). ERM recurrences arise from remnants of the ERM on the surface of the ILM, which can re-proliferate. In a histological study, a layer of collagen between the ERM and the ILM was observed, as well as areas of cellular elements adjacent to the retinal surface of the ILM. This may explain the high rate of recurrence of the ERM after its removal when ILM is not peeled (Haritoglou et al. 2004). In a large series (Shimada et al. 2009), comparing single ERM peeling and double ERM and ILM peeling, a difference arose in terms of recurrence rate, but postoperative visual acuity did not differ between the two groups. 142 eyes underwent double ERM and ILM peeling, and no one had a recurrence of the ERM. 104 eyes underwent single ERM peeling and the ERM recurred in 17 eyes (16.3 %), but only 6 eyes (5.8 %) needed a reoperation. The ILM peeled during reoperation of the 6 eyes was histologically analysed; authors detected ERM cells on the ILM and concluded that ERM recurrence arises from remnant components on the ILM that proliferate using the ILM as a scaffold. In addition, while ILM peeling during ERM surgery may reduce the risk of recurrence, it does not seem to cause adverse visual outcome. However, functional results are sometimes unsatisfactory despite successful surgical removal of the ERM.

Recently, spectral domain OCTs have recently (SD-OCT) shown that eyes with ERM can have structural abnormalities in the photoreceptors at the fovea, as suggested by the loss of photoreceptor inner segment-outer segment (IS-OS) junction line (Michalewski et al. 2007). These abnormalities were significantly correlated with poorer visual function (Inoue et al. 2011). Use of SD-OCTs have facilitated localisation and evaluation of fine foveal microstructure such as the external-limiting membrane (ELM) and cone outer segment tip (COST) (Fig. 9.1). Shimozono and co-authors analysed 49 eyes that underwent vitrectomy for ERM and evaluated the presence of alterations of ELM line, IS-OS line and COST line, on SD-OCT, and their correlation with BCVA preoperative and at 1 and 6 months postoperatively (Shimozono et al. 2012). At baseline, no eyes with altered ELM and IS-OS line were found, while 48 % of the eyes showed a disrupted COST line. The disruption of IS-OS line and COST line temporally increased at 1-month follow-up and decreased to near the baseline thereafter. At 6 months patients with integrity of IS-OS line and COST line had a significantly better BCVA than patient with alteration of IS-OS line, COST line or both. Defect diameter of IS-OS line and COST line was also significantly correlated with BCVA postoperatively. Of the 26 eyes with no defect at baseline, 14 worsened showing alteration of IS-OS line (13 eyes) or both IS-OS and COST line (1 eye) at 1 month. While of the 24 eyes with IS-OS defects at baseline, 3 eyes improved to no defects and 4 eyes worsened to a combined IS-OS and COST line defect at 1 month postoperatively. Despite its retrospective nature, this study shows

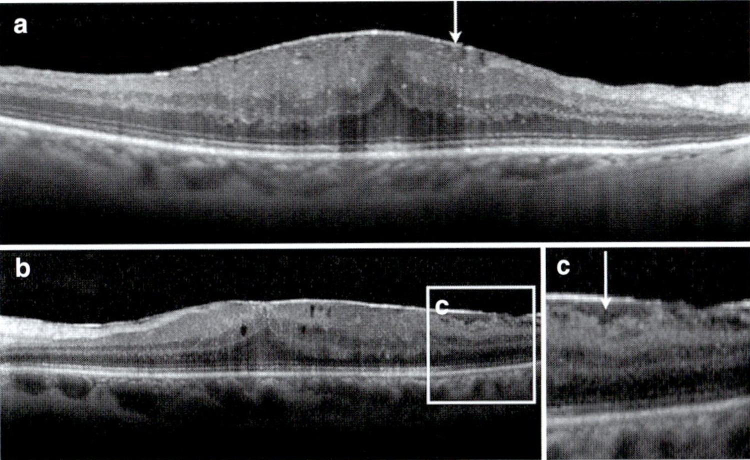

Fig. 9.2 Adherent ERM and "fibrillary changes". (**a**) SD-OCT of an ERM (*white arrow*) very adherent to the retina surface. (**b**) SD-OCT of an ERM very adherent to the retina surface with "fibrillary changes" (*white square*). (**c**) particular of (**b**). "Fibrillary changes" are visible between the ERM and the nerve fibers layer

that the status of COST line, combined with the IS-OS junction, has prognostic significance after ERM surgery. A careful examination of the outer segment status of foveal photoreceptors using OCT should be part of routine pre-operative evaluation of patients. SD-OCT with its high resolution allows better definition of the geometry of the adhesion between the membrane and the retiona and it helps to determine if membrane is focally or globally adherent to the retina surface. Recently Kim and co-authors prospectively evaluated the extent of retinal adhesion of the ERM to the retinal surface using SD-OCT and correlated their findings with the difficulty of surgically removing the ERM (Kim et al. 2012). Surgical difficulty was strongly associated with more extensive ERM adherence to the retina. Complete ERM adherence correlated with an 8.6-fold increased surgical difficulty in ERM peeling compared to focal adherence. They noted, also, a SD-OCT feature of the ERMs that correlated with surgical difficulty: the presence of, what they called, "fibrillary changes" between the ERM and the retinal nerve fibre layer (Fig. 9.2). The presence of fibrillary changes, observed by SD-OCT, correlated with a 25.5-fold increase in difficulty in completing a surgical peel, irrespective of ERM-retinal adhesion type. Authors concluded that SD-OCT analysis of ERM provides useful and valuable detailed information of the interface between the ERM and retina allowing for better surgical planning of the peeling procedure.

9.3 Macular Holes

Macular holes were first described more than 100 years ago by Knapp and Noyes (Knapp 1869; Noyes 1871). There has been a new interest in the pathogenesis and natural history of macular holes (MH) in the last two decades. With better understanding of the disease and refinements in vitreoretinal surgical techniques, macular holes are not treated successfully.

In 1991 Kelly and Wendel presented a pilot study on vitrectomy for idiopathic macular hole (Kelly and Wendel 1991). Two important surgical steps emerged from their study: removal of the cortical vitreous and peeling of the ILM. In the last years, randomised controlled trials have shown that vitrectomy associated with gas tamponade favor a very high closure rate. Gas tamponade and facedown positioning has been a central component of the treatment since its original description (Wendel et al. 1993). The "hydration theory" suggests that macular hole formation may be due to a defect in the inner retina with secondary vitreous fluid accumulation into the middle or outer retinal tissue (Tornambe 2003). If a posterior hyaloid traction (anteroposterior forces) tears the inner foveal retina, vitreous fluid soaks into this spongy layer of the macula, then dissecting deeper and accumulating also in the outer plexiform layer. As more fluid swells the macula, the hole appears to enlarge. Although water passes through the retina under normal conditions, a breech in the inner retina disrupts homeostasis. The retina swelling could be due to vitreous fluid accumulation. If the swelling resolves, the inner retinal structure reapproximates and the hole disappears. Following macular hole surgery, a gas bubble covering the holes isolates the defect from the vitreous fluid, which allows the RPE pump to quickly remove the intraretinal liquid. A mild inflammatory reaction or a small scar plugs the defect and seals the inner retina, preventing vitreous fluid from accessing the inner retinal layers. Under these circumstances, and macular holes do not reform after surgery. Intraocular tamponade is mandatory. The choice of tamponading agent and duration of postoperative facedown positioning remains a controversial subject. For most holes, a non-expansible concentration of sulphur hexafluoride and 1 week of facedown positioning optimise outcomes. Some authors have reported good results with shorter possturing, using air as tamponade or without positioning using intraocular gas or silicone oil (Park et al. 1999; Tornambe et al. 1997; Goldbaum et al. 1998). This was usually in the presence of small holes. Only 1 randomised series has been published showing a significant decrease in the success rate of MH surgery without facedown positioning, but this reduction was significant only for MH larger than 400 µm (Guillaubey et al. 2008). In 1994 a retrospective review found only a 4.8 % rate of late reopening after MH surgery, at a time when routine ILM peeling had not yet been introduced (Duker et al. 1994). While anteroposterior vitreo-macular traction is a likely mechanism for the initiation of idiopathic MHs (Gaudric et al. 1999), tangential tractions, on the retinal surface, play a role in their enlargement (Gass 1988, 1995). Proliferation of cellular components on the ILM create tangential forces around the fovea that contribute to the enlargement of the macular hole (Yooh et al. 1996; Kwok et al. 2001). For these reasons internal-limiting membrane peeling has been introduced as an additional surgical manoeuvre thereby increasing the success rate of surgery. In 2006 a retrospective study showed

that MH surgery failure mainly occured with large MHs, whereas MH smaller than 400 µm has a very high success rate, even without internal-limiting membrane peeling (Tadayoni et al. 2006). In 2000, Mester and Kuhn performed a meta-analysis of 1,654 eyes from published reports of MH surgery from 1992 to 1999 (Mester and Kuhn 2000). ILM peeling significantly improved the anatomical closure from 77 to 96 %. The study also showed a difference in functional success (2 or more Snellen lines) between the ILM peeled group (81 %) and the non-ILM peeled group (55 %). Tognetto et al. conducted a retrospective multicentre evaluation of 1,627 nonconsecutive MH operated between 1993 and 2003 (Tognetto et al. 2006). ILM was peeled in 1,100 of them. There was an overall MH closure rate of 94 % in those eyes with ILM peeling versus 89 % in eyes without ILM peeling. The authors did not find a statistically significant difference in anatomical success for stage two cases, between the two groups, but the difference was statistically significant for stages 3 and 4 holes. Funcitional outcomes were the same between the two groups. A multicentre randomised controlled trial comparing was internal-limiting membrane peeling to no peeling in patients with idiopathic stage 2 and 3 MHs showed better outcomes in the peeled group (Lois and FILMS Group 2011). 141 patients were randomised 1:1 in two groups: ILM peeling versus no peeling. Nonstatistically significant differences in distance visual acuity at 6 months were found between groups. There was a significantly higher closure rate in the ILM peeled group at 1 month with fewer numbers of reoperations performed by 6 months. Given the higher anatomic closure and lower reoperation rates in patients undergoing peeling, authors suggested that ILM peeling should be the treatment of choice for stages 2 and 3 MHs. In the same year, Tadayoni and co-workers published data from a randomised, controlled, interventional, multicentre clinical trial with the purpose to determine whether the success rate of surgery for small idiopathic macular holes (less than 400 µm) is significantly reduced if facedown positioning is

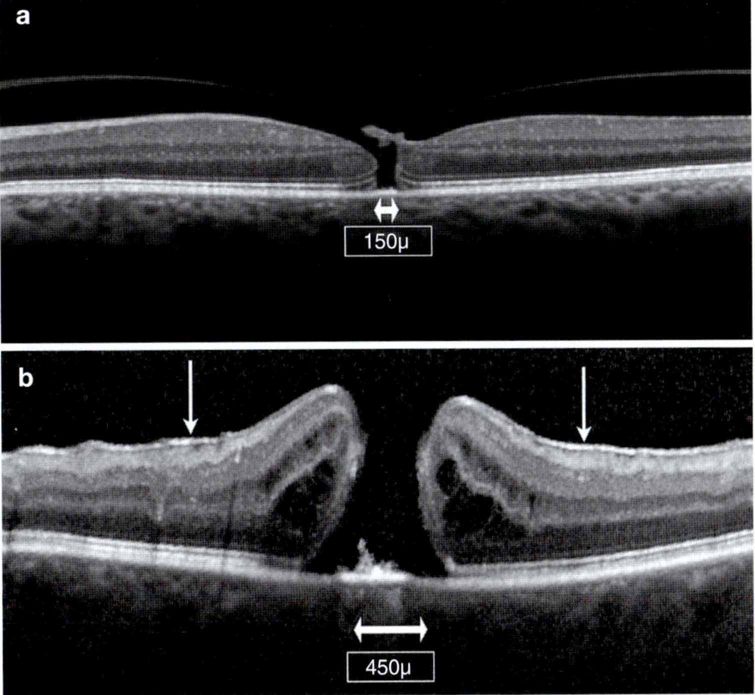

Fig. 9.3 Macular holes with and without ERMs. (**a**) SD-OCT of a small MH (150 μm of diameter) with no evidence of ERM on the retina surface. (**b**) SD-OCT of a large MH (450 μm of diameter) with evidence of an ERM (*white arrows*) on the retina surface

replaced by simply taking care to avoid the supine position (Tadayoni et al. 2011). Sixty nine patients were advised randomly to observe a strict facedown positioning for 22 of 24 h for 10 days (34 patients) or simply to avoid supine position for 10 days (35 patients). Surgical procedure included peeling of any epiretinal membrane (as determine by OCT or fundus examination), but without ILM peeling. The retinas were also not stained tamponade was with hexafluorethane. The closure rate was similar in both groups: 91.4 % in patients with minimal positioning group versus 94.1 % in the facedown positioning group (no statistical difference was found). Visual acuity at 3 months increased similarly in both groups: +10.23 letters in the group with minimal positioning group and +10.52 in the facedown positioning group. Authors concluded that the success rate of surgery for idiopathic MH of 400 μm or smaller is not significantly reduced by facedown positioning and the post-operative care can be simplified to the avoidance of a supine position for 10 days.

An appropriate treatment strategy can be devised for most if not all MH patients. A thorough preoperative examination combining fundoscopy and OCT imaging, a detailed evaluation of the health status of the patient with particular emphasis on his compliance to positioning aided by knowledge of available surgical echniques and tools (e.g. type of gas and staining) allow for such planning. Small macular holes with no evidence of an ERM (Fig. 9.3) can be treated using a gas as tamponade (C2F6 or C3F8) and avoiding supine position. But the same type of MH in a different kind of patient (e.g. a patient who needs a faster postoperative visual recovery) can be treated with a shorter acting gas and appropriate facedown positioning. In fact, the effectiveness and the need for positioning can be ascertained in the first few days after surgery by performing an OCT through the gas bubble. In the presence of an ERM (Fig. 9.3), peeling is mandatory, and combined ILM peeling reduces risk of recurrence and ensures complete removal of the ERM. In MH larger than 400 μm, peeling of any ERM and ILM should be part of the surgical procedure. In these cases positioning should be suggested and a long-standing gas chosen if surgeon is worried about compliance of the patient.

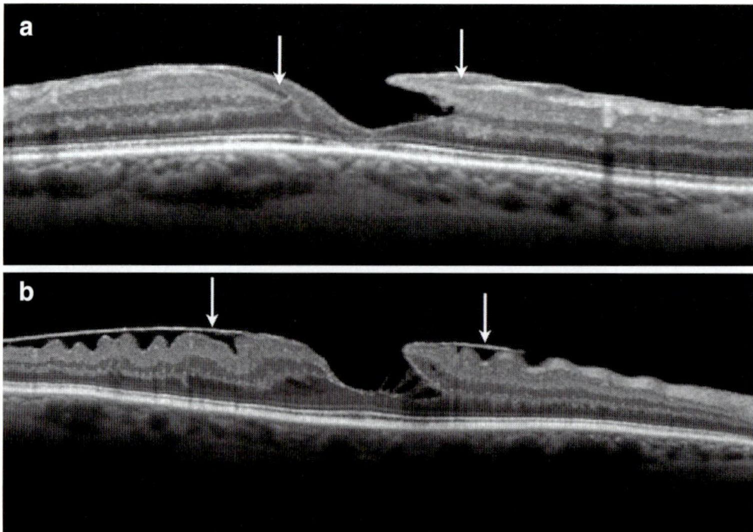

Fig. 9.4 Lamellar macular holes: normal/tractional ERM and thickened/dense ERM. (courtesy of Grazia Pertile, MD) (**a**) SD-OCT of a LMH with a thickened/dense ERM (*white arrows*). As visible the thickened/dense ERM appears on SD-OCT as a moderately-reflective material filling the space between the inner border of the ERM and the retinal nerve fiber layer. (**b**) SD-OCT of a LMH with a normal/tractional ERM (*white arrows*) that appears as a thin highly reflective line immediately anterior and separate from the retinal nerve fibers layer

9.4   Lamellar Macular Holes

Lamellar macular holes (LMHs) are a distinct clinical entity, and were originally described by Gass using biomicroscopy (Gass 1976). The diagnosis of LMH was facilitated by the introduction of OCT (Takahashi and Kishi 2000; Haouchine et al. 2004) and fundus autofluorescence (Bottoni et al. 2008), although our understanding of the pathogenesis, clinical progression and therapy of this macular defect remains controversial or incomplete. LMHs were first described as a complication of chronic cystoid macular oedema (Gass 1976). Alternatively, they might represent the result of an abortive development of a full-thickness macular hole (Gaudric et al. 1999; Haouchine et al. 2001). More recently, LMHs have been related to the contraction of an existing perifoveal epiretinal membrane-internal-limiting membrane complex (Witkin et al. 2006; Garretson et al. 2008). To distinguish LMHs from other similar macular defects, such as macular pseudoholes, Witkin and colleagues recently proposed four OCT criteria based on qualitative image analysis (Witkin et al. 2006). Criteria for the OCT diagnosis of a LMH were as follows: (1) an irregular foveal contour, (2) a break in the inner fovea, (3) a dehiscence of the inner foveal retina from the outer retina and (4) an absence of a full-thickness foveal defect with intact foveal photoreceptors. They also found that 11 eyes of the 19 examined had an ERM with an unusual appearance on OCT. They called this ERM: thickened ERM. Thickened ERM appeared on OCT as moderately reflective material filling the space between the inner border of the ERM and the retinal nerve fibre layer (Fig. 9.4). The other ERMs detected by OCT had a normal appearance: a thin highly reflective line immediately anterior and separate from the RNFL (Fig. 9.4).

LMH patients commonly have relatively good visual acuity, usually 20/40 or better. The natural course of LMHs shows that VA in these patients remains stable in almost 80 % of the cases over a follow-up period of 37.1 months (Theodossiadis 2008). Most recently, Bottoni et al. published data on evolution of LMHs using a spectral domain OCT (Bottoni et al. 2013). They prospectively examined 34 eyes of 34 patients with LMHs; the mean follow-up period was 18 months. VA did not change significantly during the follow-up period. Foveal thickness was also stable. During the baseline visit, two different types of ERM were identified: a normal ERM and a thickened ERM, as previously described by Witkin. Dividing patients into two groups, based on ERM appearance, they found that in the two groups both VA and foveal thickness remained stable during follow-up. Treatment strategies can be based on the evolution observed on natural history: vitrectomy may be indicated in LMHs showing progressive thinning within the foveal center and/or VA deterioration during the follow-up period.

Surgical treatment for LMHs is still controversial. Before 2010 surgical outcomes of only 44 patients were described in peer-reviewed literature (Hirakawa et al. 2005; Kokame and Tokuhara 2007; Witkin et al. 2006; Engler et al. 2008; Garretson et al. 2008). Thirty nine patients were vitrectomized with intraocular gas tamponade and only 5 without the use of any intraocular tamponade. Peeling of visible ERMs and of ILM was performed in all the patients. Functional results differed from one case serites to the other. More recently, in 2010, Witkin and co-authors published a retrospective evaluation on 16 patients treated with pars plana vitrectomy for LMHs (Witkin et al. 2010). There was no statistical difference between preoperative and postoperative VA. Two eyes developed a full-thickness macular hole after surgery and 6 eyes continued to have a lamellar macular defect. They concluded that vitrectomy for LMHs may not improve VA. Completely different data arose from a study by Michalewska and co-authors. The aim of their study was to report on the results of vitrectomy with ILM peeling, without gas tamponade and without postoperative positioning in 26 eyes of 26 patients with LMH confirmed on SD-OCT (Michalewska et al. 2010). Twelve months after surgery, VA improved by at least two Snellen lines in 24 eyes. The improvement was statistically significant. ERM was detected and peeled in all the cases. Lower VA was observed in patients with photoreceptor layer defects localised under the fovea based on SD-OCT findings. They concluded that vitrectomy with ERM removal and ILM peeling without gas tamponade was a useful technique in the treatment of LMHs and that poor final VA outcomes are mostly due to preoperative photoreceptor damage. Improved VA after surgery for LMHs was confirmed by Parolini and co-authors (Parolini et al. 2011). They analysed 19 eyes that underwent vitrectomy, removal of the ERM, peeling of the ILM and air tamponade, dividing patients into two groups based on ERM appearance on SD-OCT. ERM features described by Parolini et al. were similar to those described by Witkin. Postoperative VA improved significantly in patients with LMH after vitrectomy and ERM/ILM peeling. There was statistical significance in VA improvement after surgery for both types of ERM patients. ERM excised from surgery was processed for transmission electron microscopy and immunohistochemistry. They redefined the two types of ERM as "tractional" (instead of normal) and "dense" (instead of thickened) (Fig. 9.4) based upon a clinicopathologic correlation: "tractional/normal" ERM were shown to expresse by immunolabelling more frequently alpha-smooth muscle actin, as compared to present "tractional" ERMs. Since alpha-smooth muscle actin in epiretinal membranes was demonstrated to be correlated with clinical contractility, Parolini postulated that "tractional" membranes posses more potential to generate tractional forces at the retina surface than "dense" membranes. Analysing complication, 3 out of 13 patients in the "dense" ERM group developed a full-thickness macular hole after surgery. These 3 patients were successfully reoperated, but there was no improvement in VA compared to preoperative evaluation. As described by Bottoni et al. (2013), confirming data previously presented by Cereda and colleagues at an ARVO meeting (Cereda et al. 2010), "dense" membrane correlates with a thinner foveal thickness compared to "tractional" ERM. In the series of Bottoni et al. LMHs with thickened ERM had foveal thickness of 155.5 μm, while LMHs with normal ERM had

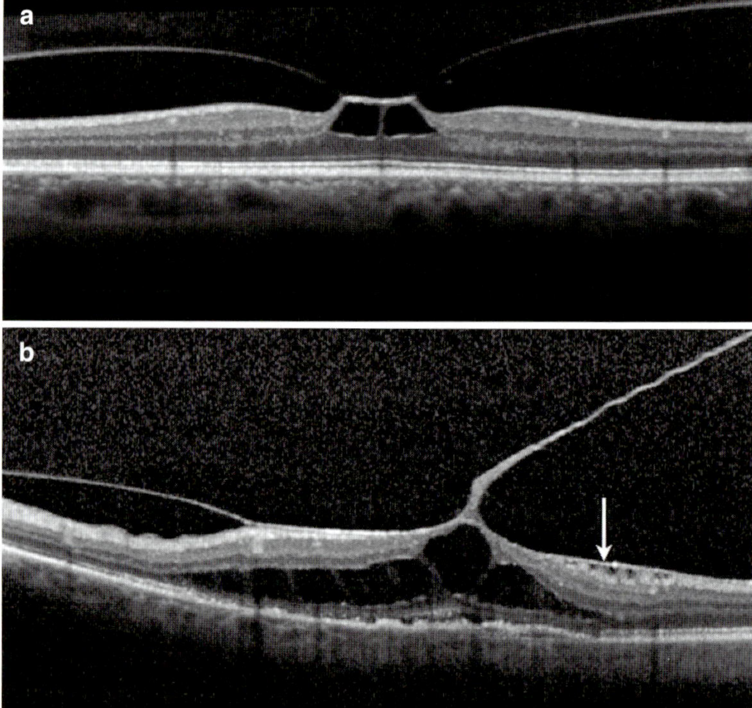

Fig. 9.5 Examples of vitreo-macular traction syndrome. (**a**) SD-OCT of a vitreo-macular traction without ERM and a focal horizontal vitreo-retina adherence. (**b**) SD-OCT of a vitreo-macular traction syndrome with concomitant ERM (*white arrow*) and a wide horizontal vitreo-retina adherence

advent of pharmacologic means of releaving traction, the appropriate choices will depend more and more on a good understanding of the pathophysiology at hand and the probability of progression. Appropriate decision making will depend on a combination of the factors discussed above, a careful evaluation of the observed changes over time, as well as the benefits of the proposed intervention.

Compliance with Ethical Requirements Dr Cereda has no conflict of interest. No animal or human studies were carried out by the author for this chapter.

References

Bottoni F, Carmassi L, Cigada M et al (2008) Diagnosis of macular pseudoholes and lamellar macular holes: is optical coherence tomography the "gold standard"? Br J Ophthalmol 92:635–639

Bottoni F, Deiro AP, Giani A et al (2013) The natural history of lamellar macular holes: a spectral domain optical coherence tomography study. Graefes Arch Clin Exp Ophthalmol 251(2):467–475

Bovey EH, Uffer S, Achache F (2004) Surgery for epimacular membrane: impact of retinal internal limiting membrane removal on functional outcome. Retina 24:728–735

Chang LK, Fine HF, Spaide RF et al (2008) Ultrastructural correlation of spectral domain optical coherence tomography findings in vitreomacular traction syndrome. Am J Ophthalmol 146:121–127

de Smet M, Gandorfer A, Stalmans P et al (2009) Microplasmin Intravitreal administration in patients with vitreomacular traction scheduled for vitrectomy. Ophthalmology 116:1349–1355

Duker JS, Wendel R, Patel AC, Puliafito CA (1994) Late re-opening of macular holes after initially successful treatment with vitreous surgery. Ophthalmology 101:1373–1378

Engler C, Schaal KB, Höh AE, Dithmar S (2008) Surgical treatment of lamellar macular hole. Ophthalmologe 105:836–839

Garretson BR, Pollack JS, Ruby AJ et al (2008) Vitrectomy for a symptomatic lamellar macular hole. Ophthalmology 115:884–886

Gass JD (1976) Lamellar macular hole: a complication of cystoid macular edema after cataract extraction. Arch Ophthalmol 94:793–800

Gass JD (1988) Idiopathic senile macular hole. Its early stages and pathogenesis. Arch Ophthalmol 106:629–639

Gass JD (1995) Reappraisal of biomicroscopic classification of stages of development of a macular hole. Am J Ophthalmol 119:752–759

Gastaud P, Bétis F, Rouhette H, Hofman P (2000) Ultrastructural findings of epimacular membrane and posterior hyaloid in vitreo-macular traction syndrome. J Fr Ophtalmol 23:587–593

Gaudric A, Haouchine B, Massin P et al (1999) Macular hole formation: new data provided by optical coherence tomography. Arch Ophthalmol 117:744–751

Goldbaum MH, McCuen BW, Hanneken AM et al (1998) Silicon oil tamponade to seal macular holes without position restrictions. Ophthalmology 105:2140–2147

Grewing R, Mester U (1996) Result of surgery for epiretinal membranes and their recurrences. Br J Ophthalmol 80:323–326

Guillaubey A, Malvitte L, Lafontaine PO et al (2008) Comparison of facedown and seated position after idiopathic macular hole surgery: a randomized clinical trial. Am J Ophthalmol 146:128–134

Haouchine B, Massin P, Gaudric A (2001) Foveal pseudocyst as the first step in macular hole formation: a prospective study by optical coherence tomography. Ophthalmology 108:15–22

Haouchine B, Massin P, Tadayoni R et al (2004) Diagnosis of macular pseudoholes and lamellar macular holes by optical coherence tomography. Am J Ophthalmol 138:732–739

Haritoglou C, Gandorfer A, Schaumberger M et al (2004) Trypan blue in macular pucker surgery: an evaluation of histology and functional outcome. Retina 24:582–590

Hikichi T, Yoshida A, Trempe CL (1995) Course of vitreomacular traction syndrome. Am J Ophthalmol 119:55–61

Hirakawa M, Uemura A, Nakano T, Sakamoto T (2005) Pars plana vitrectomy with gas tamponade for lamellar macular holes. Am J Ophthalmol 140:1154–1155

Hisatomi T, Enaida H, Sakamoto T et al (2005) A new method for comprehensive bird's eye analysis of the surgical excised internal limiting membrane. Am J Ophthalmol 139:1121–1122

Inoue M, Morita S, Watanabe Y et al (2011) Preoperative inner segment/outer segment junction in spectral-domain optical coherence tomography as a prognostic factor in epiretinal membrane surgery. Retina 31:1366–1372

Iwanoff A (1865) Beitrage zur normalen und pathologischen anatomie des auges. Graefes Arch Clin Exp Ophthalmol 11:135–170

Jaffe NS (1967) Vitreous traction at the posterior pole of the fundus due to alteration in the vitreous posterior. Trans Am Acad Ophthalmol Otolaryngol 71:642–652

Johnson MW (2005) Tractional cystoid macular edema: a subtle variant of the vitreomacular traction syndrome. Am J Ophthalmol 140:184–192

Johnson MW (2010) Posterior vitreous detachment: evolution and complications of its early stages. Am J Ophthalmol 149:371–382

Kampik A, Green WR, Michels RG, Nase PK (1980) Ultrastructural features of progressive idiopathic epiretinal membrane removed by vitreous surgery. Am J Ophthalmol 90:797–809

Kelly NE, Wendel RT (1991) Vitreous surgery for idiopathic macular holes. Result of a pilot study. Arch Ophthalmol 109:654–659

Kim JS, Chhablani J, Chan CK et al (2012) Retinal adherence and fibrillary surface changes correlate with surgical difficulty of epiretinal membrane removal. Am J Ophthalmol 153:692–697

Knapp H (1869) Uber isolirte zerreissungen der aderhaut in folge von traumen auf dem augapfel. Arch Augenheilkd 1:6–29

Kokame GT, Tokuhara KG (2007) Surgical management of inner lamellar macular hole. Ophthalmic Surg Lasers Imaging 38:61–63

Kwok AK, Li WW, Pang CP et al (2001) Indocyanine green staining and removal of internal limiting membrane in macular hole surgery: histology and outcome. Am J Ophthalmol 132:178–183

Kwok AK, Lai TY, Yuen KS (2005) Epiretinal membrane surgery with or without internal limiting membrane peeling. Clin Experiment Ophthalmol 33:379–385

Larsson J (2004) Vitrectomy in vitreomacular traction syndrome evaluated by ocular coherence tomography (OCT) retinal mapping. Acta Ophthalmol Scand 82:691–694

Lois N, Burr J, Norrie J et al (2011) Internal limiting membrane peeling versus no peeling for idiopathic full-thickness macular hole: a pragmatic randomized controlled trial. Invest Ophthalmol Vis Sci 52:1586–1592

Machemer R, Buettner H, Norton EW, Parel JM (1971) Vitrectomy: a pars plana approach. Trans Am Acad Ophthalmol Otolaryngol 75:813–820

Margherio RR, Trese MT, Margherio AR, Cartright K (1989) Surgical management of vitreomacular traction syndromes. Ophthalmology 96:1437–1445

McDonald HR, Johnson RN, Schatz H (1994) Surgical results in the vitreomacular traction syndrome. Ophthalmology 101:1397–1403

Mester V, Kuhn F (2000) Internal limiting membrane removal in the management of full-thickness macular holes. Am J Ophthalmol 129:769–777

Meyer CH, Rodrigues EB, Mennel S et al (2004) Spontaneous separation of epiretinal membrane in young subjects: personal observations and review of literature. Graefes Arch Clin Exp Ophthalmol 242:977–985

Michalewska Z, Michalewski J, Odrobina D et al (2010) Surgical treatment of lamellar macular holes. Graefes Arch Clin Exp Ophthalmol 248:1395–1400

Michalewski J, Michalewska Z, Cisiecki S, Nawrocki J (2007) Morphologically functional correlations of macular pathology connected with epiretinal membrane formation in spectral optical coherence tomography. Graefes Arch Clin Exp Ophthalmol 245:1623–1631

Noyes HD (1871) Detachment of the retina with laceration at the macular lutea. Trans Am Ophthalmol Soc 1:128–129

Odrobina D, Michalewska Z, Michalewski J et al (2011) Long-term evaluation of vitreomacular traction disorder in spectral-domain optical coherence tomography. Retina 31:324–331

Park DW, Sipperley JO, Sneed SR et al (1999) Macular hole surgery with internal-limiting membrane peeling and intravitreous air. Ophthalmology 106:1392–1397

Park DW, Dugel PU, Garda J et al (2003) Macular pucker removal with and without internal limiting membrane peeling: pilot study. Ophthalmology 110:62–64

Parolini B, Schumann RG, Cereda MG et al (2011) Lamellar macular hole: a clinicopathologic correlation of surgical excised epiretinal membranes. Invest Ophthalmol Vis Sci 52:9074–9083

Reese AB, Jones IS, Cooper WC (1970) Vitreomacular traction syndrome confirmed histologically. Am J Ophthalmol 69:975–977

Shimada H, Nakashizuka H, Hattori T et al (2009) Double staining with membrane blue G and double peeling for epiretinal membranes. Ophthalmology 116:1370–1376

Shimozono M, Oishi A, Hata M et al (2012) The significance of cone outer segment tips as a prognostic factor in epiretinal membrane surgery. Am J Ophthalmol 153:698–704

Smiddy WE, Michels RG, Glaser BM, deBustros S (1988) Vitrectomy for macular traction caused by incomplete vitreous separation. Arch Ophthalmol 106:624–628

Stalmans P, Delaey C, de Smet MD et al (2010) Intravitreal injection of microplasmin for treatment of vitreomacular adhesion: results of a prospective, randomized, sham-controlled phase II trial (the MIVI-IIT trial). Retina 30:1122–1127

Tadayoni R, Gaudric A, Haouchine B, Massin P (2006) Relationship between macular hole size and the potential benefit of internal limiting membrane peeling. Br J Ophthalmol 90:1239–1241

Tadayoni R, Vicaut E, Devin F et al (2011) A randomized controlled trial of alleviated positioning after small macular hole surgery. Ophthalmology 118:150–155

Takahashi H, Kishi S (2000) Tomographic features of a lamellar macular hole formation and a lamellar hole that progressed to a full-thickness macular hole. Am J Ophthalmol 130:677–679

Theodossiadis PG, Grigoropoulos VG, Emfietzoglou I et al (2008) Evolution of lamellar macular hole studied by optical coherence tomography. Graefes Arch Clin Exp Ophthalmol 247:13–20

Tognetto D, Grandin R, Sanguinetti G et al (2006) Internal limiting membrane removal during macular hole surgery: results of a multicentre retrospective study. Ophthalmology 113:1401–1410

Tornambe PE (2003) Macular hole genesis: the hydration theory. Retina 23:421–424

Tornambe PE, Poliner LS, Grote K (1997) Macular hole surgery without facedown positioning. A pilot study. Retina 17:179–185

Trese M, Chandler DB, Machemer R (1983) Macular Pucker. II. Ultrastructure. Graefes Arch Clin Exp Ophthalmol 221:16–26

Wendel RT, Patel AC, Kelly NE et al (1993) Vitreous surgery for macular holes. Ophthalmology 100:1671–1676

Witkin AJ, Ko TH, Fujimoto JG et al (2006) Redefining lamellar macular holes and the vitreomacular interface: an ultrahigh-resolution optical coherence tomography study. Ophthalmology 113:388–397

Witkin AJ, Castro LC, Reichel E et al (2010) Anatomic and visual outcome of vitrectomy for lamellar macular holes. Ophthalmic Surg Lasers Imaging 41:418–424

Yooh HS, Brooks HL Jr, Capone A Jr et al (1996) Ultrastructural features of tissue removed during idiopathic macular hole surgery. Am J Ophthalmol 122:67–75

Zivojnovic R, Claes C (1990) Treatment of complicated retinal detachment with proliferative vitreoretinopathy. Bull Soc Belge Ophtalmol 235:65–69

Book

Gass JDM (1987) Stereoscopic atlas of retinal diseases. Mosby, St. Louis

Online Document (No DOI Available)

Cereda MG, Mete M, Parolini B, et al (2010): Lamellar macular hole: new findings based on spectral domain-OCT and autofluorescence images. ARVO meeting abstracts. Invest Ophthalmol Vis Sci 51:1340

Morris R, Kuhn F, Witherspoon C (1990) American academy of ophthalmology annual meeting abstracts. Ophthalmology 97(Suppl):130

Pharmacologic Vitreolysis: Experimental Evidence

10

Marc D. de Smet and Aranzazu Mateo-Montoya

10.1 Introduction

Synchysis – the liquefaction of the vitreous gel and syneresis – the condensation of collagen fibers within the vitreous proper are the primary driving forces which lead to a clean separation of the posterior vitreous from the retinal surface (de Smet et al. 2013; Foos and Wheeler 1982; Sebag 2005). In line with the development of synchysis/syneresis, under physiologic conditions, a progressive attenuation of the adhesive forces between the cortical vitreous and the internal limiting membrane (ILM) develops, leading to a progressive posterior vitreous detachment (PVD). This process does not occur suddenly but rather takes months to years to complete (Johnson 2005, 2010; Larsson and Osterlin 1985; Linder 1966). The weakening of the adhesive forces between the retina and the

vitreous is a critical factor in the timing and progression of a PVD. Age-related PVD progresses normally except where firm vitreoretinal adhesions, located at the macula or the retinal periphery. With prolonged or persistent adhesions, various complications can develop such as macular hole, vitreo-macular traction, tractional diabetic macular edema, vitreous hemorrhage, and/or retina tears (Sebag 1997, 2004). Surgical solutions have been developed to treat several of these conditions, but a controlled induction of vitreous liquefaction associated with accelerated weakening of vitreoretinal adhesions is an attractive alternative, particularly since it could facilitate surgery, reduce surgical times, and possibly be used as prophylaxis (Bhisitkul 2001; Sebag 1998). Targeted pharmacologic agents capable of altering the molecular organization of the vitreous gel and the vitreoretinal interface have the potential to provide such control (Bhisitkul 2001; Sebag 1998). Several such agents have been tested over the last two decades and will be discussed further in this chapter.

Ideally, an effective vitreolytic agent must have the ability to liquefy vitreous and induce a posterior vitreous detachment. The biochemical properties of any potential vitreolytic agent include the ability to induce vitreous liquefaction and the weakening of the vitreoretinal interface. Compounds vary in their ability to affect these two components of the vitreous. They are listed in Table 10.1 based on the relative importance of their mode of action.

M.D. de Smet, MDCM, PhD, FRCSC, FRCOphth, FMH (✉)
Retina and Ocular Inflammation,
MIOS, Specialized Eye Center in Uveitis and Retina,
Avenue du Leman 32,
Lausanne, 1005, Switzerland

Vitreoretinal Surgery Unit, Clinique de Montchoisi,
Lausanne, Switzerland
e-mail: mdddesmet1@mac.com

A. Mateo-Montoya, MD, FEBO, FMH
Retina and Inflammation, MIOS,
Avenue du Leman 32, Lausanne 1005, Switzerland
e-mail: arancha.mateo@gmail.com

A. Girach, M.D. de Smet (eds.), *Diseases of the Vitreo-Macular Interface*, Essentials in Ophthalmology,
DOI 10.1007/978-3-642-40034-6_10, © Springer-Verlag Berlin Heidelberg 2014

Table 10.1 Classification of pharmacologic vitreolytic agents

Mode of action	Vitreous liquefaction	Vitreoretinal separation	Combination
Enzymatic	Hyaluronidase	Dispase	Plasmin
	Collagenase		Microplasmin
			Nattokinase
			Chondroitinase
			tPA ± plasminogen
Nonenzymatic			
		RGD peptides	

10.2 Vitreolytic Agents Causing Vitreous Liquefaction

10.2.1 Collagenase

The bacterial collagenase purified from *Clostridium histolyticum* is capable of cleaving type II collagen, abundantly present within the fibrillar network of the vitreous (Le Goff and Bishop 2008). The resultant proteolyzed fragments are soluble and subject to further degradation by nonspecific proteases. A dose-dependent liquefaction of the vitreous was observed after intravitreal incubation in rabbits. Unfortunately, it was accompanied by ILM damage and disruption of the retinal ultrastructure at doses achieving clinically significant degrees of liquefaction (O'Neill and Shea 1973). Lower doses were able to release PVR membranes in an experimental rabbit model without damaging the retina, provided the incubation time was kept under 30 min (Moorhead et al. 1983). Pilot studies in humans caused petechial hemorrhages to form on retinal fibroproliferative tissue with a 15-min exposure (Moorhead and Radtke 1985). Its narrow therapeutic window limited further development.

10.2.2 Hyaluronidase

Hyaluronidase cleaves hyaluronan and other glycosaminoglycan molecules such as chondroitin sulfate. These play an important role in maintaining the gel-like structure characteristic of the vitreous. Therefore, hyaluronidase was developed as a vitreous liquefactant. In vitro and in vivo experiments as well as a phase III clinical trial have all demonstrated its ability to accelerate clearance of vitreous hemorrhage (Foulds et al. 1985; Gottlieb et al. 1990; Kuppermann et al. 2005a, b). When injected 1–3 h prior to a standardized vitrectomy, hyaluronidase in an experimental model accelerates the extent of vitreous removal, one of the first demonstrations as a surgical adjunct (Staubach et al. 2004). Despite its impressive liquefactive abilities, hyaluronidase is limited in its capacity to induce a PVD (Hikichi et al. 2000). It is possible that its ability to liquefy vitreous combined with a limited effect on the vitreoretinal interface leaves an insufficient central support for mechanical traction on the posterior hyaloid required for a PVD to occur. Indeed, a PVD can be induced by increasing vitreoretinal traction in conjunction with the injection of hyaluronidase (Kang et al. 1995). A common adjunct has been the addition of a perfluorinated gas. Such additions could worsen existing VMA-related pathologies or precipitate their development, limiting its use in VMA pathologies (Schneider and Johnson 2011).

10.3 Vitreolytic Agents Causing Vitreoretinal Separation

10.3.1 Dispase

A neutral protease obtained from *Bacillus polymyxa*, dispase, cleaves type IV collagen and fibronectin (Stenn et al. 1989). It was first used to generate a model of PVR without the addition of exogenous cells. PVR was observed 10 or more weeks after injecting dispase intravitreally at doses of 0.01–0.50 U (Frenzel et al. 1998). Prolonged exposure leads to the release of fibroblasts, macrophages, and glial cells into the vitreous cavity.

Collagen IV and fibronectin are both found in high concentrations at the vitreoretinal interface. For this reason, attempts were made to develop dispase as an agent for enzyme-assisted vitrectomy (thereby removing the agent before it could induce PVR). For vitreolysis, higher concentrations of the enzyme were injected in the eye but with much shorter incubation periods (15–120 min) (Tezel et al. 1998). In rabbits, a dose ≤ 1 U/mL for up to 30 min or ≤ 0.05 U/mL for 1 week was found to be safe and effective in generating a PVD (Zhu et al. 2006). However, the therapeutic window is narrow, since increased dosage or time is associated with retinal and vitreous hemorrhages (Jorge et al. 2003; Wang et al. 2004). Toxicity at doses as low as 0.025 U has been observed within 1 h of intravitreal injection (Wang et al. 2004). Given safety concerns, and in particular the difficulty in defining a nontoxic therapeutic window, have severely limited the further development for human use.

10.3.2 RGD Peptide

Integrins play a critical role in extracellular matrix (ECM) adhesion and signaling (Brem et al. 1994). Binding to integrins is mediated through a specific binding motif – defined by the amino acid sequence arginine-glycine-aspartate (RGD). It is present in a large number of ECM components including laminin, fibronectin, and collagens. Synthetic RGD peptides compete for integrin binding sites, resulting in the disruption of integrin-RGD interactions and the loosening of attachments (Yang et al. 1996). For example, viper venom which contains the RGD motif inhibits RPE cell attachment to the vitreous, thus preventing RPE-induced tractional retinal detachment (Yang et al. 1996). In a rabbit model, an intravitreal injection of RGD peptide followed by a 24-h incubation leads to a higher percentage of treated eyes achieving a surgically induced PVD as compared to controls (saline injections and a nonactive RGE peptide were used as control). No toxicity was noted on electron microscopy,

clinical examination, or TUNEL apoptosis assay (Oliveira et al. 2002). No further studies have been published so far using this promising approach.

10.4 Vitreolytic Agents Causing Both Liquefaction and Vitreoretinal Separation

10.4.1 Chondroitinase

Depolymerization of various glycosaminoglycans including chondroitin sulfate, hyaluronan, and dermatan sulfate occurs under the influence of chondroitinase. The exact role of chondroitin sulfate in the vitreous remains unclear. By interacting with collagen IX, it may contribute to the vitreous structure, while others have reported that it is present along the vitreous base and the papillary margin (by immunolocalization) (Le Goff and Bishop 2008). Early preclinical experiments were promising, suggesting a complete PVD extending over the vitreous base, with a variable degree of vitreous liquefaction. Later experiments were not able to duplicate this early success and demonstrated some mild inner-limiting membrane and nerve fiber layer damage in a vitrectomy-based study (Hermel and Schrage 2007).

10.4.2 Nattokinase

Nattokinase is a serine protease produced by *Bacillus subtilis;* it has a potent fibrinolytic activity and a direct proteolytic effect on collagen. Its proteolytic target is different from plasmin enzyme, another serine protease. Hence, it acts synergistically with plasmin enzyme of which it enhances the fibrinolytic activity (Uesugi et al. 2011; Urano et al. 2001). It also inactivates inhibitors of plasminogen activator, thereby prolonging the duration of action in blood. In the vitreous, nattokinase combines a direct proteolytic effect on collagen, with an indirect effect via a plasmin-mediated vitreoretinal dehiscence. In a rabbit model, intravitreal injection resulted in PVD with bare ILM in all eyes when activity units between 0.1 and 1 were used (Takano et al. 2006). Eyes exposed to the highest concentration had discrete hemorrhages in the peripapillary retina, as well as ERG depression persisting for up to 1 week. No follow-up investigations have been reported to date. Despite a narrow therapeutic window, this particular approach alone or in combination with other vitreolytic agents may be promising.

10.4.3 Plasminogen Activators (tPA, Urokinase)

Both tPA and urokinase exert their effect indirectly by activating plasminogen and converting it into plasmin. Their nonocular use includes a number of vascular disorders including stroke, peripheral vascular occlusive disease, and symptomatic coronary artery disease. In the eye, tPA has been used to treat postsurgical fibrin formation, submacular hemorrhage, and acute retinal vein occlusion (Borillo and Regillo 2001; Kamei et al. 2000; Tameesh et al. 2004).

Their interest as vitreolytic agents stems from their well-characterized commercial formulation with an established intraocular safety record based on its use for the intraocular indications mentioned above. However, they can only work as vitreolytic agents in the presence of sufficient quantities of plasminogen. Such levels are present only in certain pathologic states associated with a blood ocular barrier breakdown (intraocular inflammation, proliferative diabetic retinopathy, intraocular hemorrhage, trauma) (Le Mer et al. 1999). Under other circumstances, sufficient intraocular levels can only be achieved by providing an exogenous source of plasminogen or by causing an iatrogenic breakdown of the ocular barrier of sufficient intensity (e.g., several applications of cryotherapy) (Hesse et al. 2000; Unal and Peyman 2000). In a rabbit model, cryopexy applied to two quadrants followed by a tPA injection 24 h later resulted in a complete PVD in all treated animals (Hesse et al. 2000). Urokinase was found to be experimentally effective when combined with an intraocular injection of plasminogen (Men et al.

2004; Unal and Peyman 2000). Preliminary studies in humans showed that tPA can cause a PVD in patients with proliferative diabetic retinopathy if injected a number of days (at least 3 days) prior to surgery (Hesse and Kroll 1999, 2000; Le Mer et al. 1999). tPA used alone in eyes with a retinal vein occlusion and traction caused a PVD in 75 % of eyes with functional improvement (Murakami et al. 2007).

While plasminogen activators have a good safety and promising efficacy profile, the therapeutic potential remains limited by the adequacy of the intraocular concentration of plasminogen. Under these circumstances, it is difficult to judge if the lack of response is due to an inadequacy of dose or lack of response. Also the variable outcome following one or more preliminary treatments reduces the appeal of this approach.

10.4.4 Plasmin Enzyme

A serine protease, plasmin plays a critical role in fibrinolysis. It has a direct effect on laminin, collagen, and possibly fibronectin (Liotta et al. 1981; Uemura et al. 2005). Through the activation of matrix metalloproteinases and elastases, its effect is extended to other extracellular matrix structures (Monea et al. 2002; Raza et al. 2000; Takano et al. 2005). In fact, these downstream activities may represent one of the important mechanisms of action of plasmin enzyme as its half-life in the vitreous cavity is less than 24 h (Verstraeten et al. 1993).

Liquefaction and vitreoretinal separation with plasmin is dependent on dose and duration of exposure (Gandorfer et al. 2001, 2002; Staubach et al. 2004; Verstraeten et al. 1993; Wang et al. 2004). In preclinical studies, the safety profile was favorable with toxicity limited to transient vitreous haze and a mild inflammatory response observed with doses up to 4U and exposures of up to 1 week (Gandorfer et al. 2001, 2002; Verstraeten et al. 1993; Wang et al. 2004). Transient ERG changes were observed in some studies. Structural damage is rarely reported, observed in one study using enucleated pig eyes (Staubach et al. 2004).

Plasmin is extremely unstable owing to rapid autolysis and inactivation by inhibitors such as α2-antiplasmin. In clinical applications, it can only be administered by activating its proenzyme – plasminogen just prior to use with tPA. As there is no approved commercial source of plasminogen, investigators have generally opted for the isolation of autologous plasminogen and its purification by affinity chromatography, a laborious and time-consuming process (Margherio et al. 1998). A disposable system allows for a more rapid isolation process taking about 30 min (Hermel et al. 2011). However, repeat preparations from a pool of human plasma using this system lead to variations in specific activity between 25.9 IU/mL and 49.8 IU/mL. Taking into account the physiologic variability in plasminogen levels among healthy individuals leads to a further increase in the possible concentration range between 21 and 55 IU/mL. In clinical use, the level of activity would not be determined following each purification procedure, as the assay is itself complicated and time consuming. The dose would be empirically determined, based on the distribution of values reported above, and aimed at obtaining an activity within the nontoxic range. It is unclear how this approach would be used in patients with systemic pathologies such as diabetes or coagulopathies where plasminogen levels deviate from normality. Several pilot studies have shown the benefit of plasmin enzyme in facilitating PVD induction at the time of surgery. Several groups have also reported an effect of plasmin enzyme on vitreous liquefaction, but the extent of this effect has not been quantified (Asami et al. 2004; Rizzo et al. 2006; Trese et al. 2000).

10.4.5 Microplasmin

A recombinant protein containing the enzymatic moiety of plasmin but not its kringles (anchor points), microplasmin is expressed and extracted as microplasminogen from a Pichia pastoris expression system. The extraction and purification steps insure sterility and a well-characterized dosage which does not differ between batches. When reconstituted from its lyophilized form and kept its citrate buffer, it retains its enzymatic activity even at room temperature for more than 2 h (Gad El Kareem et al. 2010a, b). The activity profile is similar to plasmin, acting on both laminin and fibronectin at the vitreoretinal interface, but given its significantly smaller size compared to plasmin, it can more easily diffuse through the vitreous gel (Chen et al. 2009; Gad El Kareem et al. 2010a, b).

The initial preclinical studies were carried out in enucleated pig eyes at room temperature and reported at ARVO (Valmaggia et al. 2003). To avoid artifactual separation of the vitreous from the retinal surface, a specific slow fixation technique was developed. Both dose (62.5–400 µg) and time (15–120 min) exposures were studied (de Smet et al. 2009b). These studies determined that the minimal consistently effective dose required to induce a complete PVD was 125 µg with a minimum exposure time of 1 h. No disruption of retinal cellular anatomy was seen, but serous-like retinal detachments were observed in 25 % of eyes exposed to 400 µg for 120 min. Subsequent experiments in rabbits and cats confirmed 125 µg as an effective dose (Gandorfer et al. 2004; Sakuma et al. 2005). Functional studies in rabbits showed a transient a- and b-wave reduction from day 2–7, similar to prior observations made with plasmin (Chen et al. 2008; Sakuma et al. 2005; Verstraeten et al. 1993). However, both a- and b-wave changes persisted to day 90 when eyes were injected with 250 µg.

The effect of microplasmin on the vitreous was demonstrated in two separate studies. Using dynamic light scattering, Sebag et al. was able to demonstrate a strongly dose-dependent increase in light scattering 30 min after injection of microplasmin, indicating breakdown of the vitreous structure (Sebag et al. 2007). Following injection of microplasmin close to the edge of the sclera and incubation at 37 °C for 2 h, the cornea and lens were removed and the diffusion of fluorescein dye was observed through the vitreous cavity and documented by digital photography (Gad El Kareem et al. 2010a, b). Fluorescein diffused further and more quickly in eyes injected with microplasmin > plasmin > saline. In the latter group of eyes, there was nearly no diffusion of dye within the vitreous cavity. Following a 2-h incubation, only about one-fifth of the vitreous surface was stained with fluorescein in any of the eyes injected with microplasmin, indicating that the diffusion of microplasmin and the breakdown of vitreous is a relatively slow process (Gad El Kareem et al. 2010a, b). Vitreous liquefaction can continue as long as active enzyme is present. As all serine proteases, microplasmin is a highly autolytic enzyme. In the vitreous, at therapeutic concentrations, autolytic degradation is responsible for its inactivation (Aerts et al. 2012). In porcine vitreous, starting with a dose of 125 µg, half of the activity is lost within the first 2 h. Despite this rapid autolysis, in an experimental vitreous hemorrhage model, clearance of vitreous hemorrhage occurred at similar rates and extends in hyaluronidase- and microplasmin-treated animals [submitted to *Acta Ophthalmologica* (Gad El Kareem and de Smet 2012)]. By that time, a PVD was present in all rabbits injected with 125 µg microplasmin but in none of the animals having received 55 IU of hyaluronidase. This may prove to be an interesting additional clinical target for the use of microplasmin.

Given its safety profile, microplasmin has undergone phase II and several phase III studies in vitreo-macular traction either combined with or without surgery. These clinical trials so far suggest that with a single injection, PVD induction can be expected in roughly 50 % of cases (Benz et al. 2010; de Smet et al. 2009a; Schneider and Johnson 2011; Stalmans et al. 2010).

10.5 Optimizing Vitreolysis

Preclinical research efforts in pharmacologic vitreolysis have so far been concentrated on identifying appropriate agents to cause vitreous liquefaction and/or PVD. As outlined above, several compounds have been identified which alone or in combination can achieve the desired effect. Since the ideal drug must achieve an effect without causing toxicity, it is required to operate in a fairly narrow therapeutic window. Drug combinations acting on different protein substrates might be able to enhance the rate of PVD induction while minimizing side effects. The combination of plasmin enzyme with hyaluronidase, both at the lower therapeutic range, leads to higher rates of spontaneous PVD in rabbits and diabetics rats (Wang et al. 2005; Zhi-Liang et al. 2009).

Pharmacologic vitreolysis can also be enhanced by a number of other means. For vitreolytic agents to have an effect on the vitreoretinal interface, they are required to reach the interface by diffusing through the vitreous matrix. All vitreolytic agents except urea, which was considered for a short while a few years ago, are protein based. Their surface charge, globular structures, and rate of enzymatic digestion of the vitreous matrix define their diffusion characteristics. In a model system consisting of an agarose, small-sized proteins such as lactalbumin (14kD) similar in size to microplasmin diffuse through the vitreous 25 % faster than bovine serum albumin (68kD) whose weight is similar to plasmin enzyme (Gad El Kareem et al. 2010b; Johnson et al. 1996). A similar order of difference in diffusion rates was noted between plasmin enzyme and microplasmin in vitreous (Gad El Kareem et al. 2010b). In the presence of autolytic enzymes, a determinant factor will be the site of injection. For an effect at the vitreoretinal interface, an injection should ideally be placed deep in the vitreous cavity, close to the interface. It should preferably be made within an area of liquefied vitreous as this will allow rapid diffusion to the surrounding intact vitreous matrix, a larger surface area upon which the enzyme can work. Rapid diffusion also leads to reduction in the initial concentration of enzyme, an important adjunct in reducing the autolytic process as the drug inactivation often follows second order kinetics (inactivation is based on the square of the concentration) (Aerts et al. 2012).

Finally, many of the enzymes discussed earlier not only have a direct effect on the vitreous matrix and/or interface, they also induce secondary responses by activating secondary proteolytic or inflammatory processes. RGD peptides are involved in the modulation of TGFβ, an important regulator of intraocular inflammation and the activation of macrophages (Munger and

Sheppard 2011). Plasmin and microplasmin are known to activate MMP-2 and MMP-9 which might be an important mechanism by which the activity of serine proteases are extended in the vitreous cavity beyond the residence time of the enzyme itself (Takano et al. 2005). The exact role of MMPs in this setting remains controversial (Burggraf et al. 2010).

Conclusion

Several compounds have now been identified that can act on the vitreous matrix, the vitreoretinal interface, or both. Few have been tested in humans beyond phase II, either due to a limited therapeutic window or due to less than optimal results in a clinical setting. Comparisons between compounds are hampered in the preclinical phase by the use of many different models, exposures, and analytical approaches. The modalities used to assess PVD range from clinical assessment, ultrasonography to standard histology and electron microscopy. Each approach uses different criteria to define PVD and in particular the definition of a complete PVD. Few report the presence or absence of a PVD over 360° of the retinal surface or when such a separation is finally achieved. In the case of histologic assays, the methodology used to fix the tissue greatly influences the likelihood of iatrogenic vitreous separation. To facilitate future comparisons, it would be helpful to report along with the results the limitations of the methodology used and the frequency with which in control eyes, iatrogenic events were noted. Using more than one strategy, observational, histologic, and/or analytic strategies would facilitate comparison between studies. Standardized definitions for PVD and/or liquefaction that could be applied across methodologies would greatly improve our ability to assess both new compounds and existing ones.

There is a need to better understand the molecular structure and the physiologic changes that occur both in the vitreous and at the interface with age. Furthermore, an understanding of these changes and their effect in pathologic states such as diabetes

and vascular occlusions is also lacking and yet of importance if vitreolytics are to be used some day to prevent retinal neovascularisation. Ocular vascular disease and inflammation with both reduce the function of the blood ocular barrier. Such barrier breakdown can lead to the release into the vitreous of enzymatic inhibitors that can limit the function of vitreolytic enzymes, a role in vitreolytic processes that is just beginning to be appreciated.

It is clear that many challenges face this growing discipline. However, the potential benefits from a pharmacologic approach are numerous from reduced surgical times, enhanced vision recovery, and prophylaxis from complications of vitreo-macular traction, or the presence of a vitreoretinal interface. An adequate framework for both preclinical and clinical studies will accelerate future developments.

Compliance with Ethical Requirements Prof de Smet declares to have received research grants from ThromboGenics, Inc.; received speaker's honoraria from ThromboGenics, Inc. and Alcon, Inc.; and is a consultant for ThromboGenics on preclinical studies and development. The author is also a patent holder on the ocular application of ocriplasmin. Dr Aranzazu Mateo-Montoya declares that she has no conflict of interest. No animal or human studies were carried out by the authors for this chapter.

References

Aerts F, Noppen B, Fonteyn L et al (2012) Mechanism of inactivation of ocriplasmin in porcine vitreous. Biophys Chem 165–166:30–38

Asami T, Terasaki H, Kachi S et al (2004) Ultrastructure of internal limiting membrane removed during plasmin-assisted vitrectomy from eyes with diabetic macular edema. Ophthalmology 111:231–237

Benz MS, Packo KH, Gonzalez V et al (2010) A placebo-controlled trial of microplasmin intravitreous injection to facilitate posterior vitreous detachment before vitrectomy. Ophthalmology 117:791–797

Bhisitkul RB (2001) Anticipation for enzymatic vitreolysis. Br J Ophthalmol 85:1–3

Borillo JL, Regillo CD (2001) Treatment of subretinal hemorrhages with tissue plasminogen activator. Curr Opin Ophthalmol 12:207–211

Brem RB, Robbins SG, Wilson DJ et al (1994) Immunolocalization of integrins in the human retina. Invest Ophthalmol Vis Sci 35:3466–3474

Burggraf D, Vosko MR, Schubert M et al (2010) Different therapy options protecting microvasculature after experimental cerebral ischaemia and reperfusion. Thromb Haemost 103:891–900

Chen W, Huang X, Xw M et al (2008) Enzymatic vitreolysis with recombinant microplasminogen and tissue plasminogen activator. Eye 22:300–307

Chen WL, Mo W, Sun K et al (2009) Microplasmin degrades fibronectin and laminin at vitreoretinal interface and outer retina during enzymatic vitrectomy. Curr Eye Res 34:1057–1064

de Smet MD, Gandorfer A, Stalmans P et al (2009a) Microplasmin intravitreal administration in patients with vitreomacular traction scheduled for vitrectomy: the MIVI I trial. Ophthalmology 116:1349–1355

de Smet MD, Valmaggia C, Zarrantz J et al (2009b) Microplasmin: ex vivo characterization of its activity in porcine vitreous. Invest Ophthalmol Vis Sci 50:814–819

de Smet MD, Gad Elkareem AM, Zwinderman AH (2013) The vitreous, the retinal interface in ocular health and disease. Ophthalmologica. [Epub] PMID: 23989078

Foos RY, Wheeler NC (1982) Vitreretinal juncture. Synchysis senilis and posterior vitreous detachment. Ophthalmology 89:1502–1512

Foulds WS, Allan D, Moseley H et al (1985) Effect of intravitreal hyaluronidase on the clearance of tritiated water from the vitreous of the choroid. Br J Ophthalmol 69:529–532

Frenzel E, Neely K, Walsh A et al (1998) A new model of proliferative vitreoretinopathy. Invest Ophthalmol Vis Sci 39:2157–2164

Gad Elkareem AM, de Smet MD (2012) Effect of microplasmin on the clearance of vitreous hemorrhage from an experimental model in rabbits. Acta Ophthalmol. doi: 10.1111/j.1755-3768.2012.02568.x. PMID 23025384

Gad El Kareem A, Willikens B, Vanhove M et al (2010a) Characterization of a stabilized form of microplasmin for the induction of a posterior vitreous detachment. Curr Eye Res 35:909–915

Gad El Kareem AM, Willikens B, Stassen JM et al (2010b) Differential vitreous dye diffusion following microplasmin or plasmin pre-treatment. Curr Eye Res 35:235–241

Gandorfer A, Putz E, Wege-Lüßen U et al (2001) Ultrastructure of the vitreoretinal interface following plasmin assisted vitrectomy. Br J Ophthalmol 85:6–10

Gandorfer A, Priglinger S, Schebitz K et al (2002) Vitreous morphology of plasmin treated human eyes. Am J Ophthalmol 133:156–159

Gandorfer A, Rohleder M, Sethi C et al (2004) Posterior vitreous detachment induced by microplasmin. Invest Ophthalmol Vis Sci 45:641–647

Gottlieb JL, Antoszyk A, Hatchell DL et al (1990) The safety of intravitreal hyaluronidase. A clinical and histologic study. Invest Ophthalmol Vis Sci 31:2345–2352

Hermel M, Schrage NF (2007) Efficacy of plasmin enzymes and chondroitinase ABC in creating posterior vitreous separation in the pig: a masked, placebo-controlled in vivo study. Graefes Arch Clin Exp Ophthalmol 245:399–406

Hermel M, Dailey W, Trese M et al (2011) A disposable system for rapid purification of autologous plasmin as an adjunct to vitrectomy – performance and safety profile. Graefes Arch Clin Exp Ophthalmol 249:37–46

Hesse L, Kroll P (1999) Enzymatically induced posterior vitreous detachment in proliferative diabetic retinopathy. Klin Monbl Augenheilkd 214:84–89

Hesse L, Kroll P (2000) TPA-assisted vitrectomy for proliferative diabetic retinopathy. Retina 20:317–318

Hesse L, Nebeling B, Schroeder B et al (2000) Induction of posterior vitreous detachment in rabbits by intravitreal injection of tissue plasminogen activator following cryopexy. Exp Eye Res 70:31–39

Hikichi T, Kado M, Yoshida A (2000) Intravitreal injection of hyaluronidase cannot induce posterior vitreous detachment in the rabbit. Retina 20:195–198

Johnson MW (2005) Perifoveal vitreous detachment and its macular complications. Trans Am Ophthalmol Soc 103:537–567

Johnson MW (2010) Posterior vitreous detachment: evolution and complications of its early stages. Am J Ophthalmol 149:371–382

Johnson EM, Berk DA, Jain RK et al (1996) Hindered diffusion in agarose gels: test of effective medium model. Biophys J 70:1017–1026

Jorge R, Oyamaguchi EK, Cardillo JA et al (2003) Intravitreal injection of dispase causes retinal hemorrhages in rabbit and human eyes. Curr Eye Res 26:107–112

Kamei M, Estafanous M, Lewis H (2000) Tissue plasminogen activator in the treatment of vitreoretinal diseases. Semin Ophthalmol 15:44–50

Kang SW, Hyung SM, Choi MY et al (1995) Induction of vitreolysis and vitreous detachment with hyaluronidase and perfluoropropane gas. Korean J Ophthalmol 9:69–78

Kuppermann BD, Thomas EL, de Smet MD et al (2005a) Safety results of two phase III trials of an intravitreous injection of highly purified ovine Hyaluronidase (Vitrase) for the management of vitreous hemorrhage. Am J Ophthalmol 140:585–587

Kuppermann BD, Thomas EL, de Smet MD et al (2005b) Pooled efficacy results from two multinational randomized controlled clinical trials of a single intravitreous injection of highly purified ovine hyaluronidase (Vitrase) for the management of vitreous hemorrhage. Am J Ophthalmol 140:573–584

Larsson L, Osterlin S (1985) Posterior vitreous detachment. A combined clinical and physicochemical study. Graefes Arch Clin Exp Ophthalmol 223:92–95

Le Goff MM, Bishop PN (2008) Adult vitreous structure and postnatal changes. Eye 22:1214–1222

Le Mer Y, Korobelnik JF, Morel C et al (1999) TPA-assisted vitrectomy for proliferative diabetic retinopathy. Results of a double-masked, multicenter trial. Retina 19:378–382

Linder B (1966) Acute posterior vitreous detachment and its retinal complications. Acta Ophthalmol Suppl 87:5–107

Liotta LA, Goldfarb RH, Brundage R et al (1981) Effect of plasminogen activator (urokinase), plasmin, and thrombin on glycoprotein and collagenous components of basement membrane. Cancer Res 41: 4629–4636

Margherio AR, Margherio RR, Hartzer M et al (1998) Plasmin enzyme-assisted vitrectomy in traumatic pediatric macular holes. Ophthalmology 105: 1617–1620

Men G, Peyman GA, Genaidy M et al (2004) The role of recombinant lysine-plasminogen and recombinant urokinase and sulfur hexafluoride combination in inducing posterior vitreous detachment. Retina 24:199–209

Monea S, Lehti K, Keski-Oja J et al (2002) Plasmin activates pro-matrix metalloproteinase-2 with a membrane-type 1 matrix metalloproteinase-dependent mechanism. J Cell Physiol 192:160–170

Moorhead LC, Radtke N (1985) Enzyme-assisted vitrectomy with bacterial collagenase. Pilot human studies. Retina 5:98–100

Moorhead LC, Chu HH, Garcia CA (1983) Enzyme-assisted vitrectomy with bacterial collagenase. Time course and toxicity studies. Arch Ophthalmol 101: 265–274

Munger JS, Sheppard D (2011) Cross talk among TGF-beta signaling pathways, integrins, and the extracellular matrix. Cold Spring Harb Perspect Biol 3:a005017

Murakami T, Takagi H, Ohashi H et al (2007) Role of posterior vitreous detachment induced by intravitreal tissue plasminogen activator in macular edema with central retinal vein occlusion. Retina 27:1031–1037

O'Neill R, Shea M (1973) The effects of bacterial collagenase in rabbit vitreous. Can J Ophthalmol 8:366–370

Oliveira LB, Meyer CH, Kumar J et al (2002) RGD peptide-assisted vitrectomy to facilitate induction of a posterior vitreous detachment: a new principle in pharmacological vitreolysis. Curr Eye Res 25:333–340

Raza SL, Nehring LC, Shapiro SD et al (2000) Proteinase-activated receptor-1 regulation of macrophages (MMP-12) secretion by serine proteinases. J Biol Chem 52:41243–41250

Rizzo SM, Pellegrini GP, Benocci FM et al (2006) Autologous plasmin for pharmacologic vitreolysis prepared 1 hour before surgery. Retina 26:792–796

Sakuma T, Tanaka M, Mizota A et al (2005) Safety of in vivo pharmacologic vitreolysis with recombinant microplasmin in rabbit eyes. Invest Ophthalmol Vis Sci 46:3295–3299

Schneider EW, Johnson MW (2011) Emerging nonsurgical methods for the treatment of vitreomacular adhesion: a review. Clin Ophthalmol 5:1151–1165

Sebag J (1997) Classifying posterior vitreous detachment: a new way to look at the invisible. Br J Ophthalmol 81:521

Sebag J (1998) Pharmacologic vitreolysis. Retina 18:1–3

Sebag J (2004) Anomalous posterior vitreous detachment: a unifying concept in vitreo-retinal disease. Graefes Arch Clin Exp Ophthalmol 242:690–698

Sebag J (2005) Molecular biology of pharmacologic vitreolysis. Trans Am Ophthalmol Soc 103:473–494

Sebag J, Ansari R, Suh K (2007) Pharmacologic vitreolysis with microplasmin increases vitreous diffusion coefficients. Graefes Arch Clin Exp Ophthalmol 245:576–580

Stalmans P, de Laey C, de Smet M et al (2010) Intravitreal injection of microplasmin for treatment of vitreomacular adhesion: results of a prospective, randomized, sham-controlled phase II trial (the MIVI-IIT trial). Retina 30:1122–1127

Staubach F, Nober V, Janknecht P (2004) Enzyme-assisted vitrectomy in enucleated pig eyes: a comparison of hyaluronidase, chondroitinase, and plasmin. Curr Eye Res 29:261–268

Stenn KS, Link R, Moellmann G et al (1989) Dispase, a neutral protease from *Bacillus polymyxa*, is a powerful fibronectinase and type IV collagenase. J Invest Dermatol 93:287–290

Takano A, Hirata A, Inomata Y et al (2005) Intravitreal plasmin injection activates endogenous matrix metalloproteinase-2 in rabbit and human vitreous. Am J Ophthalmol 140:654–660

Takano A, Hirata A, Ogasawara K et al (2006) Posterior vitreous detachment induced by nattokinase (subtilisin NAT): a novel enzyme for pharmacologic vitreolysis. Invest Ophthalmol Vis Sci 47:2075–2079

Tameesh MK, Lakhanpal RR, Fujii GY et al (2004) Retinal vein cannulation with prolonged infusion of tissue plasminogen activator (tPA) for the treatment of experimental retinal vein occlusion in dogs. Arch Ophthalmol 138:829–839

Tezel TH, Del Priore LV, Kaplan HJ (1998) Posterior vitreous detachment with dispase. Retina 18:7–15

Trese MT, Williams GA, Hartzer MK (2000) A new approach to stage 3 macular holes. Ophthalmology 107:1607–1611

Uemura A, Nakamura M, Kachi S et al (2005) Effect of plasmin on laminin and fibronectin during plasmin-assisted vitrectomy. Arch Ophthalmol 123: 209–213

Uesugi Y, Usuki H, Iwabuchi M et al (2011) Highly potent fibrinolytic serine protease from streptomyces. Enzyme Microb Technol 48:7–12

Unal M, Peyman GA (2000) The efficacy of plasminogen-urokinase combination in inducing posterior vitreous detachment. Retina 20:69–75

Urano T, Ihara H, Umemura K et al (2001) The profibrinolytic enzyme subtilisin NAT purified from Bacillus subtilis Cleaves and inactivates plasminogen activator inhibitor type 1. J Biol Chem 276: 24690–24696

Valmaggia C, Willekens B, de Smet MD (2003) Microplasmin induced vitreolysis in porcine eyes. Invest Ophthalmol Vis Sci 44:E Abstract 3050

Verstraeten TC, Chapman C, Hartzer M et al (1993) Pharmacologic induction of posterior vitreous detachment in the rabbit. Arch Ophthalmol 111: 849–854

Wang F, Wang Z, Sun X et al (2004) Safety and efficacy of dispase and plasmin in pharmacologic vitreolysis. Invest Ophthalmol Vis Sci 45:3286–3290

Wang Z-LM, Zhang XM, Xu XM et al (2005) PVD following plasmin but not hyaluronidase: implications for combination pharmacologic vitreolysis therapy. Retina 25:38–43

Yang CH, Huang TF, Liu KR et al (1996) Inhibition of retinal pigment epithelial cell-induced tractional retinal detachment by disintegrins, a group of Arg-Gly-Asp-containing peptides from viper venom. Invest Ophthalmol Vis Sci 37:843–854

Zhi-Liang W, Wo-Dong S, Min L et al (2009) Pharmacologic vitreolysis with plasmin and hyaluronidase in diabetic rats. Retina 29:269–274

Zhu D, Chen H, Xu X (2006) Effects of intravitreal dispase on vitreoretinal interface in rabbits. Curr Eye Res 31:935–946

Pharmacologic Vitreolysis: Clinical Trial Data

11

Steve Pakola and Julia A. Haller

11.1 Introduction

11.1.1 Why Pharmacologic Vitreolysis?

Recognition of the importance of vitreo-macular interface pathology in various retinal disorders has grown in recent years (Sebag 2004; Johnson 2010), in large part due to the remarkable advances in imaging of the vitreoretinal interface made possible by optical coherence tomography. In particular, anomalous PVD with remaining vitreo-macular adhesion (VMA) is increasingly recognized, as well as its pathologic sequelae of vitreo-macular traction and macular hole. Vitreo-macular adhesion has also been implicated in the exacerbation of other retinal disorders, including retinal vein occlusion, diabetic retinopathy, and age-related macular degeneration (Avunduk et al 1997; Nasrallah et al 1988; Akiba et al 1990; Haller et al 2010; Krebs et al 2007; Mojana et al 2008; Robison et al 2009).

Patients with VMT and macular hole have a poor prognosis if left untreated. Most untreated eyes undergo a further decrease in vision and in some cases progressive complications (Hikichi et al. 1995). In patients with symptomatic VMA who underwent vitrectomy, greater improvement in visual acuity was observed in eyes with better preoperative visual acuity and shorter duration of symptoms (Melberg et al. 1995; Sonmez et al. 2008). Thus, the data suggest that earlier treatment of this spectrum of disorders may help achieve better visual outcome. Nevertheless, the invasiveness, risks, expense, and inconvenience of vitrectomy typically limit its use to patients with advanced disease (Guillaubey et al. 2007; Ramkissoon et al. 2010; Rizzo et al. 2010; Banker et al. 1997; Cheng et al. 2001; Freeman et al. 1997; Recchia et al. 2010). Therefore, patients often remain untreated until the condition progressively worsens to a point that warrants surgery.

The goal of therapy for symptomatic VMA and related conditions is to relieve traction on the macula thereby resolving the underlying condition with subsequent functional improvement. The only treatment option available currently to achieve this goal is surgery (vitrectomy). A minimally invasive, less traumatic, and well-tolerated pharmacological treatment option would represent a significant advance in care. It is for these reasons that the retina community has over the last two decades advanced pharmacologic vitreolysis as a potential treatment option for addressing diseases of the vitreo-macular interface like symptomatic VMA as well as for treatment of other retinal diseases where vitreo-macular interface pathology may play an exacerbating role. Pharmacologic vitreolysis refers to the

S. Pakola, MD (✉)
Clinical Development, Amakem NV,
15 Lewis Rd, Irvington, NY 10533, USA
e-mail: steve.pakola@amakem.com

J.A. Haller, MD
Wills Eye Institute, 840 Walnut Street, Suite 1510,
Philadelphia, PA 19107, USA
e-mail: jhaller@willseye.org

A. Girach, M.D. de Smet (eds.), *Diseases of the Vitreo-Macular Interface*, Essentials in Ophthalmology,
DOI 10.1007/978-3-642-40034-6_11, © Springer-Verlag Berlin Heidelberg 2014

Table 11.1 Pharmacologic vitreolytic agents

Agent	Liquefactant/ interfactant	Mechanism of action	Stage of development
Hyaluronidase	+/−	Cleavage of hyaluronan	Clinical testing (Phase 3)/not being developed for this indication
Collagenase	+/−	Cleavage of type II collagen	Clinical testing with observed toxicities/discontinued
Dispase	−/+	Cleavage of type IV collagen and fibronectin	Preclinical testing/discontinued
Vitreosolve	+/+	Urea-based compound	Discontinued during Phase 3
Chondroitinase	+/+	Depolymerization of chondroitin sulfate	Preclinical testing/discontinued
Nattokinase	+/+	Enhance plasminogen activators and inactivating plasmin activator inhibitor	Preclinical testing
Plasminogen activator	+/+	Indirect activation of plasmin	Clinical testing (pilot studies)
Plasmin	+/+	Cleavage of glycoproteins including laminin, fibronectin, and collagen	Clinical testing (pilot studies)
Ocriplasmin	+/+	Laminin, fibronectin, and collagen	Clinical testing (Phase 3)

intravitreal administration of an agent to induce vitreous liquefaction and/or vitreoretinal separation (Sebag 1998 and 2009). Although there is currently no approved pharmacologic treatment available for diseases of the vitreo-macular interface, encouraging clinical results have been reported in recent years.

11.1.2 Targets for Pharmacologic Vitreolysis

Enzymes that target one or more of the substrates that make up the vitreous and or the "molecular glue" at the vitreoretinal interface have received the most attention in the search for a safe and effective pharmacologic vitreolytic agent. Although this search has been pursued in earnest for over two decades, most molecules evaluated have not been successful either because of lack of efficacy or because of toxicity due to lack of specificity. The most relevant substrates for vitreoretinal adhesion have been reported to be fibronectin and laminin (Sebag 2005; Le Goff and Bishop 2008). Plasmin-based products, which are known to have activity against fibronectin and laminin as well as collagen, have achieved the most success in clinical development to date. This has included pilot clinical trials evaluating tissue plasminogen activator (tPA) and autologous plasmin enzyme

and more recently Phase 2 and Phase 3 clinical trials evaluating ocriplasmin (a recombinantly produced, truncated form of human plasmin with retained protease activity).

The current characterization of pharmacologic vitreolytic agents is based on whether they achieve vitreous liquefaction (liquefactants) and/ or vitreoretinal separation (interfactants), with ideal agents demonstrating both characteristics. Agents that have been evaluated preclinically are included in Table 11.1. This chapter will review the available clinical results for those agents that have been evaluated for treatment of vitreoretinal interface disorders as well as retinal disorders that may be exacerbated by vitreoretinal interface pathology.

11.1.3 Indications Explored in Clinical Trials

Because pathology at the vitreoretinal interface is known to play a role in various vitreoretinal disorders, there are several potential approaches/ patient populations that can be considered for evaluation of safety and efficacy of molecules that target pathology at the vitreoretinal interface. Initially, the field of pharmacologic vitreolysis focused on the goal of an adjunct to vitrectomy that would facilitate vitreous separation intraoperatively, in order to make surgery faster, easier, and/or decrease the risk of complications. Accordingly, the early trials discussed in this chapter evaluate the use of these agents administered prior to planned vitrectomy in conditions including vitreo-macular traction and macular hole and in pediatric vitrectomy settings including retinopathy of prematurity (ROP). However, encouraging results in some of these trials raised the possibility that such agents may also be considered for pharmacologic treatment thereby potentially resolving the underlying condition *without* the need for surgical intervention and the associated burden of treatment and complications associated with surgery. Such pharmacologic treatment indications can be broken down into those where the vitreoretinal interface disorder is the underlying condition to be treated (namely, vitreo-macular traction with or without associated macular hole, referred to as symptomatic vitreo-macular adhesion) and those conditions where vitreoretinal interface pathology may play an exacerbating role, e.g., retinal vein occlusion, diabetic retinopathy, and age-related macular degeneration.

11.2 Clinical Results

11.2.1 Collagenase

Highly purified bacterial collagenase (clostridiopeptidase A) resulted in dose-dependent liquefaction of the vitreous after intravitreal injection in rabbits, although it also showed some internal limiting membrane damage in this animal model (O'Neill and Shea 1973). A pilot study of collagenase as an adjunct to vitrectomy in humans showed promising effects without side effects (Moorhead and Radtke 1985). In this study, six patients with dense intravitreal fibroproliferative tissue associated with retinopathy of prematurity, diabetic retinopathy, or proliferative vitreoretinopathy were injected with bacterial collagenase intraoperatively 15 min prior to removal by irrigation/aspiration, with no side effects, including no retinal hemorrhage. However, in a separate study, retinal hemorrhages attributed to digestion

of the retinal vasculature were observed (Takahashi et al. 1993). No further study results have been reported since these findings.

11.2.2 Hyaluronidase

While hyaluronan and collagen are the main components of the vitreous (Bishop 2000; Sebag 2005; Le Goff and Bishop 2008), hyaluronan does not play a role in vitreoretinal adhesion. Therefore, it is not surprising that in preclinical testing, hyaluronidase has shown more effect in terms of vitreous liquefaction (Narayanan and Kuppermann 2009; Gottlieb et al. 1990) than for PVD induction (Wang et al. 2005; Hikichi et al. 2000). Consistent with these findings, clinical assessment of Vitrase® (commercial name of highly purified ovine hyaluronidase produced by ISTA Pharmaceuticals, Irvine, USA) has focused on treatment of vitreous hemorrhage as opposed to vitreoretinal interface disorders.

The Phase 3 program for treatment of vitreous hemorrhage involved two studies utilizing a placebo-controlled, double-masked design in which 1,362 subjects were randomized to intravitreal hyaluronidase at doses of 7.5, 55, and 75 IU or placebo. The patients enrolled in the North American study were assigned to one of four treatment arms (saline injection, 7.5, 55, or 75 IU Vitrase injection), while the patients treated in the second study outside North America were assigned to one of three treatment arms (saline injection, 55 or 75 IU Vitrase injection). In the pooled efficacy analysis across 1,125 patients who received the 55 or 75 IU doses or saline placebo in the two studies, statistical significance was reached as early as months 1 and 2 for the 55 IU dose group for the primary endpoint (clearance of hemorrhage sufficient to see the underlying pathology and completion of treatment when indicated) (Kuppermann 2005a). The most common observed toxicity was acute, self-limited iritis with a dose-dependent incidence (Kuppermann 2005b). Assessment of PVD or other aspects of the vitreoretinal interface was not performed in the Phase 3 studies. While Vitrase is approved for use as a spreading agent, the FDA after review of the Phase 3 trial results for treatment of vitreous hemorrhage did not approve the drug for this indication.

In a separate Phase 2 study performed in Mexico, 60 NPDR patients were randomly assigned to one of four treatment groups. A single intravitreous injection was given to one eye of each patient: saline (0.05 ml), Vitrase (75 IU, 0.05 ml), SF6 gas (0.3 ml), or Vitrase plus SF6 gas 4 weeks later. A higher proportion of eyes treated with Vitrase had stable ETDRS retinopathy scores as compared to saline. The percent of eyes with a complete PVD and stable ETDRS scores was highest in the eyes treated with Vitrase, although the small sample size and lack of OCT assessment to evaluate the status of the vitreoretinal interface limit interpretation of these results. The results were presented at ARVO (Kuppermann et al. 2002) but have not been published.

11.2.3 Vitreosolve

Vitreosolve is a urea-based compound initially developed by Vitreoretinal Technologies Inc. (Irvine, CA) for treatment of patients with diabetic retinopathy with attached vitreous. The goal of treatment is to induce a PVD and thereby decrease progression of diabetic retinopathy. After Phase 2 development supported that vitreosolve was generally well tolerated and had potential to induce PVD, a Phase 3 trial intended to enroll 400 patients was initiated. Development was subsequently discontinued after an interim analysis suggested the trial would not meet its primary endpoint.

11.2.4 Tissue Plasminogen Activator

Tissue plasminogen activator (tPA) has been used as an alternative to autologous plasmin due to its ability to convert intraocular plasminogen to plasmin. Tissue plasminogen activator is commercially available as an approved product for treatment of intravascular thrombotic disorders (including acute myocardial infarction and

acute stroke), and safety data exist for intraocular use for other disorders (Kamei et al. 2000). Unfortunately, because tPA acts indirectly via activation of endogenous plasminogen into plasmin, efficacy is dependent on available plasminogen at the site of intended effect, in this case the vitreous and the vitreoretinal interface. Perhaps because plasminogen is present in much lower concentrations in these locations than in the systemic circulation, preclinical results have shown less compelling evidence of PVD induction compared to that observed with plasmin or microplasmin. The potential for greater efficacy in disease states where there is blood-retinal barrier breakdown that may allow for greater plasminogen concentrations in the vitreous/vitreoretinal interface (e.g., proliferative vitreoretinopathy, retinal vein occlusion, and diabetic retinopathy) remains a possibility. When 25 μg of tissue plasminogen activator was injected 15 min prior to vitrectomy in patients with proliferative vitreoretinopathy this was shown to facilitate the procedure (Hesse et al. 1995). However, in another study in patients with proliferative diabetic retinopathy using the same dose of tissue plasminogen activator compared to buffered salt solution (BSS) injected 15 min prior to vitrectomy in a double-masked fashion, no difference was found between the treatment group and control (Le Mer et al. 1999). A separate study evaluated tPA injection without subsequent vitrectomy in patients with macular edema secondary to CRVO (Murakami et al. 2007). While this retrospective study only included 21 eyes with attached vitreous prior to tPA administration, tPA was associated with PVD induction in these patients and tPA induction of PVD did correlate with improvement in macular thickness and VA. A more recent prospective randomized trial in 27 patients with refractory DME comparing intravitreal tPA administration to no treatment showed a higher rate of PVD induction in patients administered with tPA, but no effect on either macular thickness or VA was observed (Abrishami et al. 2011).

Larger controlled studies would be needed to confirm a potential effect of tPA in any of these treatment settings. Given the unpredictable amount of substrate plasminogen that would be present even in these disease states where blood-retinal barrier breakdown exists, exploration of a plasmin-based product that does not rely on local endogenous plasminogen concentrations would be more amenable to evaluation in these treatment settings.

11.2.5 Plasmin

Plasmin is a nonspecific serine protease that mediates intravascular fibrinolysis. In addition to fibrin, it acts on several glycoproteins including laminin and fibronectin which are present at the vitreoretinal interface (Liotta et al. 1981; Uemura et al. 2005; Li et al. 2002). Numerous preclinical studies support plasmin's ability to induce PVD (Li et al. 2002; Verstraeten et al. 1993; Hikichi et al. 1999; Gandorfer et al. 2001). A drawback of plasmin is that it is not available for clinical use and its use is further complicated by the fact that plasmin is unstable. Therefore, clinical application requires activation of its proenzyme, plasminogen which in its turn is also not commercially available for human use. Investigators therefore have to go through the time-consuming and costly process of autologous plasminogen isolation from a patient's own blood which subsequently has to be converted in vitro to plasmin, also referred to as autologous plasmin enzyme, and then purified and tested to confirm sterility (Margherio et al. 1998). Several human pilot studies have been performed using this technique with doses ranging from 0.03 to 2 U in different vitreoretinal interface disorders. Because of the strong VMA in pediatric patients, several studies have been performed in this age group, notably in the surgical treatment of traumatic macular holes (Margherio et al. 1998; Wu et al. 2007) and stage 5 retinopathy of prematurity (Tsukahara et al. 2007; Wu et al. 2008). Plasmin was generally well tolerated and showed suggestions of favorable effect in terms of surgical outcomes; however, these studies were generally uncontrolled and so interpretation is limited. Plasmin also showed encouraging results as an adjunct to vitrectomy in adults in small uncontrolled studies in macular holes

(Trese et al. 2000; Sakuma et al. 2005a), diabetic macular edema (Azzolini et al. 2004; Sakuma et al. 2006), and proliferative diabetic retinopathy (Hirata et al. 2007).

Several small, uncontrolled studies support the potential of intravitreal plasmin injection without vitrectomy to induce PVD in patients with macular edema secondary to retinal vein occlusion, and that PVD induction is associated with decreased macular edema and improved VA (Udaondo et al. 2011; Sakuma et al. 2010). Larger controlled studies are needed to assess the potential benefit of plasmin for the treatment of this and other retinal disorders. However, due to the practical limitations and quality assurance issues of individualized preparation of autologous plasmin enzyme, more definitive trials to evaluate the safety and efficacy of this product for regulatory purposes is not foreseen.

11.2.6 Ocriplasmin (Generic Name of Molecule Microplasmin)

Ocriplasmin is a recombinant truncated form of human plasmin obtained from microplasminogen produced in a Pichia pastoris expression system by recombinant DNA technology (Gandorfer et al. 2004). It contains the catalytic domain of plasmin (Gad Elkareem et al. 2010). Therefore, the shortcomings of autologous plasmin are addressed by this recombinant protein that has improved stability with retained catalytic properties, e.g., towards laminin, fibronectin, and collagen at the vitreoretinal interface. Initial investigations on pig and human postmortem eyes revealed achievement of complete PVD as demonstrated by bare internal limiting membrane similar to that previously demonstrated with plasmin (Gandorfer et al. 2004). Subsequent in vivo studies in felines and rabbits confirmed these findings (Gandorfer et al. 2004).

Based on the encouraging preclinical findings, a series of clinical trials was undertaken collectively referred to as the Microplasmin Intravitreal Injection (MIVI) trials. Dose response was evaluated in one uncontrolled Phase I/IIa study (MIVI-I) and in two controlled Phase 2 studies

(MIVI-IIT and MIV-IIII) (de Smet et al. 2009a, b; Stalmans et al. 2010; Benz et al. 2010) using intravitreal ocriplasmin doses of 25–175 μg. In addition, a study in patients with diabetic macular edema was conducted (MIVI-II DME), but results of this study have not been published yet. All ocriplasmin doses were well tolerated. The 125 μg dose was associated with optimal efficacy with no additional benefit observed with the 175 μg dose. Therefore, ocriplasmin 125 μg was selected for further evaluation in the Phase 3 pivotal studies.

The Phase 3 trials (referred to as the MIVI-TRUST studies) evaluated the efficacy and safety of 125 μg of intravitreal ocriplasmin versus placebo in the treatment of patients with symptomatic VMA (Haller 2011; Dugel and MIVI-TRUST Study Group 2011). It involved two nearly identical multicenter, randomized, placebo-controlled, double-masked studies (MIVI-006 and MIVI-007 trials). The primary endpoint was resolution of VMA at day 28, determined by central reading center optical coherence tomography (OCT) evaluation. In total, 652 eyes were treated. Results demonstrated highly statistically significant improved rate of pharmacological resolution of VMA in ocriplasmin group compared to placebo. Statistical analysis of the combined data demonstrated VMA resolution in 26.5 % of ocriplasmin-injected patients compared to 10.1 % in placebo ($p<0.001$). Induction of total PVD was also more prevalent in ocriplasmin-injected patients (13.4 %) compared with placebo-injected patients ($p<0.001$). Nonsurgical closure of macular holes by day 28 occurred in 40.6 % of ocriplasmin-injected eyes compared to 10.6 % in placebo-injected eyes ($p=0.004$). Ocriplasmin-injected patients exhibited a higher incidence of 2-lines (23.7 %) and 3-lines (9.7 %) improvement in best corrected visual acuity without vitrectomy during the study compared with placebo-injected patients ($p<0.001$). Based on these results, a Biologics License Application and a Marketing Authorization Application has been submitted to the FDA and EMA, respectively, for use of ocriplasmin for the treatment of patients with symptomatic vitreo-macular adhesion including macular hole.

Conclusion

Vitreoretinal interface pathology is an increasingly well-documented causative or exacerbating factor in numerous vitreoretinal disorders. Anomalous PVD with vitreo-macular adhesion is culpable in the development of vitreo-macular traction and macular hole, and potentially plays an exacerbating role in numerous other diseases including epiretinal membrane, retinal vein occlusion, diabetic retinopathy, and age-related macular degeneration. There has been interest in pharmacologically targeting the vitreoretinal interface to treat these diseases. These efforts have begun to bear fruit, as evidenced by clinically meaningful results from trials of plasmin-based products, most notably ocriplasmin. Further discovery, preclinical, and clinical work is needed to further elucidate the role of the vitreoretinal interface in retinal disease and to improve efficacy rates in the treatment of these sight-threatening conditions.

Compliance with Ethical Requirements Dr. Haller consults for the following companies: ThromboGenics, Second Sight, Advanced Cell Technology, Merck, Regeneron, KalVista, Genentech, and Alcon. She has equity in OptiMedica. Dr. Pakola is a former employee of ThromboGenics Inc and has no other conflicts of interest. No animal or human studies were carried out by the authors for this article.

References

Abrishami M, Moosavi MN, Shoeibi N, Hosseinpoor SS (2011) Intravitreal tissue plasminogen activator to treat refractory diabetic macular edema by induction of posterior vitreous detachment. Retina 31(10):2065–2070

Akiba J, Arzabe CW, Trempe CL (1990) Posterior vitreous detachment and neovascularization in diabetic retinopathy. Ophthalmology 97:889–891

Avunduk A, Cetinkaya K, Kapicioglu Z, Kaya C (1997) The effect of posterior vitreous detachment on the prognosis of branch retinal vein occlusion. Acta Ophthalmol Scand 75:441–442

Azzolini C, D'Angelo A, Maestranzi G et al (2004) Intrasurgical plasmin enzyme in diabetic macular edema. Am J Ophthalmol 138:560–566

Banker AS, Freeman WR, Kim JW, Munguia D, Azen SP (1997) Vision-threatening complications of surgery for full-thickness macular holes. Vitrectomy for Macular Hole Study Group. Ophthalmology 104:1442–1453

Benz MS, Packo KH, Gonzalez V, Pakola S, Bezner D, Haller JA, Schwartz SD (2010) A placebo-controlled trial of microplasmin intravitreous injection to facilitate posterior vitreous detachment before vitrectomy. Ophthalmology 117:791–797

Bishop PN (2000) Structural macromolecules and supramolecular organisation of the vitreous gel. Prog Retin Eye Res 19:323–344

Cheng L, Azen SP, El-Bradey MH et al (2001) Duration of vitrectomy and postoperative cataract in the vitrectomy for macular hole study. Am J Ophthalmol 132:881–887

de Smet MD, Gandorfer A, Stalmans P, Veckeneer M, Ferone E, Pakola S, Kampik A (2009a) Microplasmin intravitreal administration in patients with vitreomacular traction scheduled for vitrectomy: the MIVI I trial. Ophthalmology 116:1349–1355

de Smet MD, Valmaggia C, Zarranz-Ventura J, Willekens B (2009b) Microplasmin: ex vivo characterization of its activity in porcine vitreous. Invest Ophthalmol Vis Sci 50:814–819

Dugel PU, MIVI-TRUST Study Group (2011) A single injection of ocriplasmin for the treatment of symptomatic vitreomacular adhesion (sVMA): results of the Phase 3 MIVI-TRUST Program. Invest Ophthalmol Vis Sci 52(Suppl):6628

Freeman WR, Azen SP, Kim JW, El-Haig W, Mishell DR, Bailey I (1997) Vitrectomy for the treatment of full-thickness stage 3 or 4 macular holes. Results of a multicentered randomized clinical trial. The Vitrectomy for Treatment of Macular Hole Study Group. Arch Ophthalmol 115:11–21

Gad Elkareem AM, Willekens B, Vanhove M, Noppen B, Stassen JM, de Smet MD (2010) Characterization of a stabilized form of microplasmin for the induction of posterior vitreous detachment. Curr Eye Res 35:909–915

Gandorfer A, Putz E, Welge-Lussen U, Gruterich M, Ulbig M, Kampik A (2001) Ultrastructure of the vitreoretinal interface following plasmin assisted vitrectomy. Br J Ophthalmol 85:6–10

Gandorfer A, Rohleder M, Sethi C et al (2004) Posterior vitreous detachment induced by microplasmin. Invest Ophthalmol Vis Sci 45:641–647

Gottlieb JL, Antoszyk AN, Hatchell DL, Saloupis P (1990) The safety of intravitreal hyaluronidase. A clinical and histologic study. Invest Ophthalmol Vis Sci 31:2345–2352

Guillaubey A, Malvitte L, Lafontaine PO et al (2007) Incidence of retinal detachment after macular surgery: a retrospective study of 634 cases. Br J Ophthalmol 91:1327–1330

Haller JA (2011) The vitreomacular interface and ocriplasmin 2011. Presented at Retina 2011, Orlando, FL, USA, 21–22 October 2011, pp 1–2. http://www.aao.org/pdf/Retina-2011-Syllabus.pdf. Assessed 24 Feb 2012

Haller JA, Qin H, Apte RS et al (2010) Vitrectomy outcomes in eyes with diabetic macular edema and vitreomacular traction. Ophthalmology 117:1087–1093

Hesse L, Chofflet J, Kroll P (1995) Tissue plasminogen activator as a biochemical adjuvant in vitrectomy for proliferative vitreoretinopathy. Ger J Ophthalmol 4:323–327

Hikichi T, Yoshida A, Trempe CL (1995) Course of vitreomacular traction syndrome. Am J Ophthalmol 119:55–61

Hikichi T, Yanagiya N, Kado M, Akiba J, Yoshida A (1999) Posterior vitreous detachment induced by injection of plasmin and sulfur hexafluoride in the rabbit vitreous. Retina 19:55–58

Hikichi T, Kado M, Yoshida A (2000) Intravitreal injection of hyaluronidase cannot induce posterior vitreous detachment in the rabbit. Retina 20:195–198

Hirata A, Takano A, Inomata Y, Yonemura N, Sagara N, Tanihara H (2007) Plasmin-assisted vitrectomy for management of proliferative membrane in proliferative diabetic retinopathy: a pilot study. Retina 27:1074–1078

Johnson MW (2010) Posterior vitreous detachment: evolution and complications of its early stages. Am J Ophthalmol 149:371–382

Kamei M, Estafanous M, Lewis H (2000) Tissue plasminogen activator in the treatment of vitreoretinal diseases. Semin Ophthalmol 15:44–50

Krebs I, Brannath W, Glittenberg C et al (2007) Posterior vitreomacular adhesion: a potential risk factor for exudative age-related macular degeneration? Am J Ophthalmol 144:741–746

Kuppermann BD, Quiroz Mercado H, Graue-Wiechers F, Thomas EL, Calvillo PN, Grillone LR (2002) Effect of intravitreous hyaluronidase (Vitrase®) on progression of diabetic retinopathy in humans. Invest Ophthalmol Vis Sci, ARVO, May 5, 2002

Kuppermann BD, Thomas EL, de Smet MD, Grillone LR for the vitrase for vitreous hemorrhage study groups (2005a) Pooled efficacy results from two multinational randomized controlled clinical trials of a single intravitreous injection of highly purified ovine hyaluronidase (Vitrase) for the management of vitreous hemorrhage. Am J Ophthalmol 140:573–584

Kuppermann BD, Thomas EL, de Smet MD, Grillone LR for the vitrase for vitreous hemorrhage study groups (2005b) Safety results of two Phase 3 trials of an intravitreous injection of highly purified ovine hyaluronidase (Vitrase) for the management of vitreous hemorrhage. Am J Ophthalmol 140:585–597

Le Goff MM, Bishop PN (2008) Adult vitreous structure and postnatal changes. Eye (Lond) 22:1214–1222

Le Mer Y, Korobelnik JF, Morel C, Ullern M, Berrod JP (1999) TPA-assisted vitrectomy for proliferative diabetic retinopathy: results of a double-masked, multicenter trial. Retina 19:378–382

Li X, Shi X, Fan J (2002) Posterior vitreous detachment with plasmin in the isolated human eye. Graefes Arch Clin Exp Ophthalmol 240:56–62

Liotta LA, Goldfarb RH, Brundage R, Siegal GP, Terranova V, Garbisa S (1981) Effect of plasminogen activator (urokinase), plasmin, and thrombin on glycoprotein and collagenous components of basement membrane. Cancer Res 41:4629–4636

Margherio AR, Margherio RR, Hartzer M, Trese MT, Williams GA, Ferrone PJ (1998) Plasmin enzyme-assisted vitrectomy in traumatic pediatric macular holes. Ophthalmology 105:1617–1620

Melberg NS, Williams DF, Balles MW et al (1995) Vitrectomy for vitreomacular traction syndrome with macular detachment. Retina 15:192–197

Mojana F, Cheng L, Bartsch DU et al (2008) The role of abnormal vitreomacular adhesion in age-related macular degeneration: spectral optical coherence tomography and surgical results. Am J Ophthalmol 146:218–227

Moorhead LC, Radtke N (1985) Enzyme-assisted vitrectomy with bacterial collagenase. Pilot human studies. Retina 5:98–100

Murakami T, Takagi H, Obashi H et al (2007) Role of posterior vitreous detachment induced by intravitreal tissue plasminogen activator in macular edema with central retinal artery occlusion. Retina 27(8):1031–1037

Narayanan R, Kuppermann BD (2009) Hyaluronidase for pharmacologic vitreolysis. Dev Ophthalmol 44:20–25

Nasrallah F, Jalkh A, Van Coppenolle F (1988) The role of the vitreous in diabetic macular edema. Ophthalmology 95:1335–1339

O'Neill R, Shea M (1973) The effects of bacterial collagenase in rabbit vitreous. Can J Ophthalmol 8:366–370

Ramkissoon YD, Aslam SA, Shah SP, Wong SC, Sullivan PM (2010) Risk of iatrogenic peripheral retinal breaks in 20-G pars plana vitrectomy. Ophthalmology 117:1825–1830

Recchia FM, Scott IU, Brown GC, Brown MM, Ho AC, Ip MS (2010) Small-gauge pars plana vitrectomy: a report by the American Academy of Ophthalmology. Ophthalmology 117:1851–1857

Rizzo S, Belting C, Genovesi-Ebert F, Di Bartolo E (2010) Incidence of retinal detachment after small-incision, sutureless pars plana vitrectomy compared with conventional 20-gauge vitrectomy in macular hole and epiretinal membrane surgery. Retina 30:1065–1071

Robison CD, Krebs I, Binder S et al (2009) Vitreomacular adhesion in active and end-stage age- related macular degeneration. Am J Ophthalmol 148:79–82

Sakuma T, Tanaka M, Inoue M, Mizota A, Souri M, Ichinose A (2005a) Efficacy of autologous plasmin for idiopathic macular hole surgery. Eur J Ophthalmol 15:787–794

Sakuma T, Tanaka M, Mizota A, Inoue J, Pakola S (2005b) Safety of in vivo pharmacologic vitreolysis with recombinant microplasmin in rabbit eyes. Invest Ophthalmol Vis Sci 46:3295–3299

Sakuma T, Tanaka M, Inoue J, Mizota A, Souri M, Ichinose A (2006) Use of autologous plasmin during vitrectomy for diabetic maculopathy. Eur J Ophthalmol 16:138–140

Sakuma T, Mizota A, Inoue J, Tanaka M (2010) Intravitreal injection of autologous plasmin enzyme for macular edema associated with branch retinal vein occlusion. Am J Ophthalmol 150(6):876–882

Sebag J (1998) Pharmacologic vitreolysis. Retina 18:1–3

Sebag J (2004) Anomalous posterior vitreous detachment: a unifying concept in vitreo-retinal disease. Graefes Arch Clin Exp Ophthalmol 242:690–698

Sebag J (2005) Molecular biology of pharmacologic vitreolysis. Trans Am Ophthalmol Soc 103:473–494

Sebag J (2009) Pharmacologic vitreolysis – premise and promise of the first decade. Retina 29:871–874

Sonmez K, Capone A Jr, Trese MT, Williams GA (2008) Vitreomacular traction syndrome: impact of anatomical configuration on anatomical and visual outcomes. Retina 28:1207–1214

Stalmans P, Delaey C, de Smet MD, van Dijkman E, Pakola S (2010) Intravitreal injection of microplasmin for treatment of vitreomacular adhesion: results of a prospective, randomized, sham-controlled phase II trial (the MIVI-IIT trial). Retina 30:1122–1127

Takahashi K, Nakagawa M, Ninomiya H et al (1993) Enzyme-assisted vitrectomy with collagenase. Jpn J Clin Ophthalmol 47:802–803

Trese MT, Williams GA, Hartzer MK (2000) A new approach to stage 3 macular holes. Ophthalmology 107:1607–1611

Tsukahara Y, Honda S, Imai H et al (2007) Autologous plasmin-assisted vitrectomy for stage 5 retinopathy of prematurity: a preliminary trial. Am J Ophthalmol 144:139–141

Udaondo P, Diaz-Llopis M, Garcia-Delpech S, Salom D, Romero FJ (2011) Intravitreal plasmin without vitrectomy for macular edema secondary to branch retinal vein occlusion. Arch Ophthalmol 129:283–287

Uemura A, Nakamura M, Kachi S et al (2005) Effect of plasmin on laminin and fibronectin during plasmin-assisted vitrectomy. Arch Ophthalmol 123:209–213

Verstraeten TC, Chapman C, Hartzer M, Winkler BS, Trese MT, Williams GA (1993) Pharmacologic induction of posterior vitreous detachment in the rabbit. Arch Ophthalmol 111:849–854

Wang ZL, Zhang X, Xu X, Sun XD, Wang F (2005) PVD following plasmin but not hyaluronidase: implications for combination pharmacologic vitreolysis therapy. Retina 25:38–43

Wu WC, Drenser KA, Trese MT, Williams GA, Capone A (2007) Pediatric traumatic macular hole: results of autologous plasmin enzyme-assisted vitrectomy. Am J Ophthalmol 144:668–672

Wu W-C, Drenser KA, Lai M, Capone A, Trese MT (2008) Plasmin enzyme-assisted vitrectomy for primary and reoperated eyes with stage 5 retinopathy of prematurity. Retina 28(Suppl 3):S75–S80

Marc D. de Smet and Baruch D. Kuppermann

12.1 Introduction

In this book, we have summarized our knowledge about the vitreoretinal interface, our ability to visualize the various states of physiologic and pathologic changes, and the nascent area of pharmacologic therapy. Over the past two decades, thanks to the development of ever more performing optical coherent tomography, we have gained an increasing understanding of the role played by the vitreous in macular and retinal diseases (Gad El Kareem et al 2013; Johnson 2012; Johnson 2013). Age-related posterior vitreous detachment (PVD), long thought to be an acute event with a precipitous onset and rapid progression, is now recognized as a slow process often taking years, extending first superiorly before extending inferiorly to the peripheral retina. A significant number of disorders commonly treated by vitreoretinal surgeons are exacerbated by deviations in this physiologic process, either through abnormal adhesions or anomalous vitreous separation (Johnson 2012; Schneider and Johnson 2011; Sebag 2008; Wang et al 2009).

Among the treatment option available, pharmacologic vitreolysis offers the possibility of intervening before substantial vision loss and the need for a surgical intervention, thereby minimizing inherent risks and cost. So far, only ocriplasmin has been approved for this indication. The clinical development program showed that after a single intravitreal injection, vitreo-macular separation occurred more often in eyes treated with ocriplasmin than in placebo-injected eyes (26.5 % vs 10.1 %) (de Smet et al 2009; Stalmans et al 2010, 2012). However, these results indicate that there is still a significant margin for improvement before pharmacologic vitreolysis can be considered successful in the majority of injected patients. In parallel with attempts to develop better vitreolytic agents with a similar or better safety profile than ocriplasmin, there is room for other approaches including alternate delivery procedures, repeat injections, or combination therapies (Sebag 2007). While impending or small-sized macular holes, vitreo-macular traction in the absence of an epiretinal membrane, were seen as the most promising indicators of success in the ocriplasmin development program, the use of a vitreolytic agent as prophylaxis against vitreoretinal pathologies requires further exploration.

M.D. de Smet, MDCM, PhD, FRCSC, FRCOphth,
FMH (✉)
Retina and Ocular Inflammation, MIOS,
Specialized Eye Center in Uveitis and Retina,
Avenue du Leman 32, Lausanne, 1005, Switzerland

Vitreoretinal Surgery Unit,
Clinique de Montchoisi, Lausanne, Switzerland
e-mail: mdddesmet1@mac.com

B.D. Kuppermann, MD, PhD
Gavin Herbert Eye Institute, University of California,
Irvine, CA, USA

A. Girach, M.D. de Smet (eds.), *Diseases of the Vitreo-Macular Interface*, Essentials in Ophthalmology,
DOI 10.1007/978-3-642-40034-6_12, © Springer-Verlag Berlin Heidelberg 2014

12.2 Optimizating Nonsurgical Vitreo-macular Separation

12.2.1 Nonpharmacologic Means

It has long been known that intravitreal gas injection can induce a PVD and potentially treat vitreo-macular disorders (Chan et al 1995; Rodrigues et al 2013; Thresher et al 1984). In 1995, Chan and associates first published the use of an intravitreal gas bubble to treat macular holes (Chan et al 1995). In their series, 10 of 11 impending holes responded to treatment, but 2 stage 3 holes failed to close. In a retrospective series, Rodrigues et al reported a 40 % resolution of vitreo-macular traction with the use of C3F8 gas at 1 month and 60 % at 6 months. The most successful cases were patients with small areas of adhesion, limited retinal elevation, and low vitreous face reflectivity (Rodrigues et al 2013). Ochoa-Contreras and associates reported the successful induction of a PVD in 12 diabetic eyes (Ochoa-Contreras et al 2000). While these eyes did not have vitreo-macular traction, the contralateral eyes did not develop a PVD during a 2-year follow-up. Diabetes may predispose eyes to PVD by allowing the release of proteases after disruption of the blood ocular barrier (Gao et al 2008). Gas therefore in the appropriate patient population, either alone or in combination with pharmacologic means, may be a successful strategy to increase the likelihood of releasing VMT. Similar results may be possible in other conditions leading a weakened blood ocular barrier such as inflammatory syndromes or trauma.

12.2.2 Optimizing Drug Delivery

A number of published reports have demonstrated that serine proteases cause a decrease in vitreous viscosity (Gad El Kareem et al 2010; Sebag et al 2007). This effect is time and dose dependent. Partial vitreous liquefaction facilitates diffusion of the enzyme through the vitreous cavity, both extending its vitreolytic activity and increasing the surface area which can be reached by the enzyme before autolytic catalysis eliminates its activity (Aerts et al 2012; de Smet et al 2012). Since the posterior vitreous, particularly the macular area, is generally the target of vitreoretinal adhesions of interest, an injection within the mid-vitreous or deeper would increase the enzymatic activity close to the intended site of action.

Reflux of injected drugs along the needle track is a common problem observed in 36–46 % of patients receiving a 0.05 mL injection of an anti-VEGF (Rodrigues et al 2007; Usman Saeed et al 2011). Though the refluxed fluid in many cases is not the active compound (Boon et al 2008), with serine proteases, the absence of an excess amount of effective drug at the time of injection requires that reflux is kept to a minimum. Certain steps such as a bevelled injection, use of a Honan balloon, deep needle placement, or removing fluid from the anterior chamber can reduce the severity of reflux by 50–100 % (Hong and Jee 2012; Hubschman et al 2010; Rodrigues et al 2011). Needle gauge and type also may influence the ability to deliver a drug to the vitreous cavity as well as determine the accuracy of the delivered quantity (Hubschman et al 2010). Important variations exist with currently available needles, particularly with regard to the residual volume and the quality of the needle's workmanship. Novel needle designs may help to direct the injected drug more homogeneously in the deep vitreous and minimize reflux (Asami et al 2012).

Such refinements in delivery will be important to maximize the effect of enzyme targeting the vitreous.

12.2.3 Combination Treatments and Alternative Pharmacologies

In addition to physical or physicochemical means of improving vitreous separation, it may be possible to act on the PVD process itself. The physiologic separation of the posterior hyaloid calls for the cleavage of bonds between the posterior hyaloid and the basement membranes of Mueller cells followed by the separation of the posterior hyaloid which occurs under the combined influence of a fluid shift from the adjacent vitreous into the retrohyaloidal space and a posteroanterior contraction of the vitreous body induced by condensation of the vitreous collagen fibrils (Gad El Kareem et al 2013; Sebag 2008). In an experimental rabbit model, PVD induction took 4 or more weeks to develop following an injection of ocriplasmin in mid-vitreous. Plasmin is also effective at creating a cleavage plane and at causing significant synchysis (Gad El Kareem et al 2010). However, in a diabetic rat model, combining plasmin with hyaluronidase leads to a more consistent PVD induction than could be achieved with either drug alone (Wang et al 2005; Zhi-Liang et al 2009). In this model, PVD induction appeared to occur within one week of injection. While the authors speculated that hyaluronidase facilitated the diffusion of plasmin to the interface between the retina and the vitreous, an alternative explanation suggests that the hyaluronidase was a more effective agent at causing vitreous liquefaction—a prerequisite for an efficient PVD. Combining two drugs, one effective on the vitreous proper and the other on the interface, may lead to synergy with regard to PVD induction. The timing between the two injections—simultaneous or separating the two by several hours or days—would require further elucidation. A combination between a serine protease and nonenzymatic disruption of the vitreous might be worth exploring, as it would minimize the breakdown of the enzymatic protein co-injected with a serine protease (Schneider and Johnson 2011).

12.3 Additional Targets for Pharmacologic Treatment

While pharmacological vitreolysis as a result of the ocriplasmin development program has centered on the release of symptomatic vitreomacular traction leading in some cases to the resolution of macular holes (de Smet et al 2009; Stalmans et al 2012), other clinical entities are worth considering.

Clinical observations dating back to the 1980s and 1990s have shown that a PVD is likely beneficial in preventing retinal neovascularization (Akiba et al 1990; Ono et al 2005; Tagawa et al 1986; Takahashi et al 1981). Indeed, the posterior hyaloid may act as a scaffold for new vessel formation as well as favor the development of macular edema (Akiba et al 1990; Faulborn and Bowald 1985; NasrAllah et al 1988) A meta-analysis of data published up to early 2012 showed that the presence of a partial PVD versus a complete PVD was highly likely to be associated with proliferative diabetic retinopathy (PDR) with an odds ratio of 186 (Gad El Kareem et al 2013). In this setting, a complete PVD versus none leads to a lowered odds ratio of 0.097. Both did not cross the midline. The protection offered by a complete PVD suggests that the prophylactic induction of a PVD, if complete, may be desirable in patients at risk for PDR. A prospective clinical trial in patients with high-risk systemic and ocular signs would be desirable, given the pandemic nature of diabetes today.

A PVD in the setting of a retinal vein occlusion also leads to a "protective effect," with an odds ratio of 0.06 in regard to neovascularization. Less significant effects were noted for age-related macular degeneration and macular edema of various causes. In these diseases, while vitreous traction or oxygenation may contribute to a better outcome, many other factors appear to play a role. Thus, it may be more difficult to demonstrate a beneficial effect of a prophylactic pharmacologic vitreolysis in this setting.

12.4 Improving Visualization

In the previous section, we alluded to the use of vitreolysis as a prophylactic agent. We also indicated that a partial PVD might under certain circumstances make matters worse than not having a PVD at all. Adequate visualization of the interface is therefore important. Current technologies were assessed in a number of studies (Barak et al 2012). The presence of a partial PVD can be assessed equally well by ultrasound and OCT, though finer details of the retinal attachment are better seen on OCT (Mojana et al 2010). In the MIVI Trust study, both time domain and spectral domain OCTs gave readers a similar ability to detect vitreoretinal interface abnormalities, but the ease of interpretation was greatest with spectral domain (Folgar et al 2012). To detect pathology on the retinal surface, such as epiretinal membranes, spectral domain is superior with significantly higher detection rates possible, particularly when assessed by physicians rather than trained readers (Falkner-Radler et al 2010; Folgar et al 2012). Since the presence of surface membranes may reduce the ability of pharmacologic agents to cause a PVD, their identification on preoperative images is important.

Current systems are capable of identifying the presence of vitreous adhesion to the retinal surface when at least one area of separation between the retina and the vitreous is present (within the detection limits of the instrument being used) (De Croos et al. 2012). Complete presence of a PVD or its complete absence can only be currently assessed by ultrasound. While ideal to give a general overview of the vitreous, ultrasound's ability to image the posterior retinal surface is limited using current technology. One can expect these limitations to be overcome by use of linear array transducers. OCT signal at the vitreoretinal interface will improve with faster scanning modes, particularly for structures that are not well adherent to the retinal surface and when the scanning strategy calls for signal averaging. However, it may also be improved in the current machine by using novel approaches—noise reduction algorithms adapted to the specific scanning technologies, differential visualization algorithms for vitreous and retina, or the use of combined scanning modes (Barteselli et al. 2013), novel segmentation strategies based potentially on the RPE signal rather than the retinal vitreous interface so that the latter is better imaged. Imaging can also be enhanced by context. C scanning or horizontal scans have the advantage of allowing one to visualize a larger area, correlating with alterations visible along vascular landmarks or on a broader area of the retinal surface (Tammewar et al 2009).

Conclusion

Better understanding the role of vitreous and vitreo-macular traction has led to the development of novel treatment strategies. Those that are now available require optimization. The exact context in which they can and will be used needs to be further defined. This optimization would be facilitated by adequate imaging, required not only to image traction but

also to the interface pathologies that could interfere with a successful intervention. Along the line, appropriate scanning algorithms and a common terminology for interface structures both normal and abnormal will be required.

Compliance with Ethical Requirements Porf de Smet declares to have received research grants from ThromboGenics and received speaker's honoraria from ThromboGenics, Inc and Alcon, Inc and is a consultant for ThromboGenics on preclinical studies and development. The author is also a patent holder on the ocular application of ocriplasmin. Dr. Kuppermann was a consultant and clinical investigator for ISTA Pharmaceuticals and a clinical investigator and is currently a consultant for ThromboGenics and Alcon. He has received speaker's honoraria from ThromboGenics and Alcon. Dr. Kuppermann has no other relevant disclosures in the field of vitreolysis. No animal or human studies were carried out by the authors for this article.

References

Aerts F, Noppen B, Fonteyn L et al (2012) Mechanism of inactivation of ocriplasmin in porcine vitreous. Biophys Chem 165–166:30–38. doi:10.1016/j.bpc.2012.03.002

Akiba J, Arzabe CW, Trempe CL (1990) Posterior vitreous detachment and neovascularization in diabetic retinopathy. Ophthalmology 97:889–891

Asami T, Wong SC, Mitchell PC et al (2012) A novel quadraport needle with improved intravitreal drug dispersion. Retina 32:1222–1225

Barak Y, Ihnen MA, Schaal S (2012) Spectral domain optical coherence tomography in the diagnosis and management of vitreoretinal interface pathologies. J Ophthalmol 2012:876472. doi:10.1155/2012/876472

Barteselli G, Bartsch DU, El-Emam S et al (2013) Combined depth imaging technique on spectral-domain optical coherence tomography. Am J Ophthalmol 155:727–732. doi:10.1016/j.ajo.2012.10.019

Boon C, Crama N, Klevering B et al (2008) Reflux after intravitreal injection of bevacizumab. Ophthalmology 115:1268

Chan CK, Wessels IF, Friedrichsen EJ (1995) Treatment of idiopathic macular holes by induced posterior vitreous detachment. Ophthalmology 102:757–767

De Croos FC, Toth CA, Folgar FA et al (2012) Characterization of vitreoretinal interface disorders using OCT in the interventional phase 3 trials of ocriplasmin. Invest Ophthalmol Vis Sci 53:6504–6511. doi:10.1167/iovs.12-10370

de Smet MD, Gandorfer A, Stalmans P et al (2009) Microplasmin intravitreal administration in patients with vitreomacular traction scheduled for vitrectomy: the MIVI I trial. Ophthalmology 116:1349–1355

de Smet MD, Gad El Kareem A, Zwinderman AH (2013) The vitreous, the retinal interface in ocular health and disease. Ophthalmologica in press. doi: 10.1159/000353447

de Smet MD, Jonckx B, Vanhove M et al (2012) Pharmacokinetics of ocriplasmin in vitreous. Invest Ophthalmol Vis Sci 53:8208–8213. doi:10.1167/iovs.12-10148

Falkner-Radler CI, Glittenberg C, Hagen S et al (2010) Spectral-domain optical coherence tomography for monitoring epiretinal membrane surgery. Ophthalmology 117:798–805. doi:10.1016/j.ophtha.2009.08.034

Faulborn J, Bowald S (1985) Microproliferations in proliferative diabetic retinopathy and their relationship to the vitreous: corresponding light and electron microscopic studies. Graefes Arch Clin Exp Ophthalmol 223:130–138

Folgar FA, Toth CA, DeCroos FC et al (2012) Assessment of retinal morphology with spectral and time domain OCT in the phase III trials of enzymatic vitreolysis. Invest Ophthalmol Vis Sci 53:7395–7401. doi:10.1167/iovs.12-10379

Gad El Kareem AM, Willikens B, Stassen JM et al (2010) Differential vitreous dye diffusion following microplasmin or plasmin pre-treatment. Curr Eye Res 35:235–241

Gad El Kareem A, Zwinderman AH, Mateo-Montoya A, et al (2013) The vitreous and its retinal interface in ocular health and disease. Ophthalmologica (in press)

Gao BB, Chen X, Timothy N et al (2008) Characterization of the vitreous proteome in diabetes without diabetic retinopathy and diabetes with proliferative diabetic retinopathy. J Proteome Res 7:2516–2525

Hong SW, Jee D (2012) Effect of the honan intraocular pressure reducer to prevent vitreous reflux after intravitreal bevacizumab injection. Eur J Ophthalmol 22:615–619

Hubschman JP, Coffee RE, Bourges JL et al (2010) Experimental model of intravitreal injection techniques. Retina 30:167–173

Johnson MW (2012) Posterior vitreous detachment. Evolution and role in macular disease. Retina 32:S174–S178

Johnson MW (2013) How should we release vitreomacular traction: surgically, pharmacologically, or pneumatically? Am J Ophthalmol 155:203–205.e1. doi:10.1016/j.ajo.2012.10.016

Mojana F, Kozak I, Oster SF et al (2010) Observations by spectral-domain optical coherence tomography combined with simultaneous scanning laser ophthalmoscopy: imaging of the vitreous. Am J Ophthalmol 149:641–650. doi:10.1016/j.ajo.2009.11.016

NasrAllah FP, Jalkh AE, Van Coppenolle F et al (1988) The role of the vitreous in diabetic macular edema. Ophthalmology 95:1335–1339

Ochoa-Contreras E, Delsol-Coronado L, Buitrago ME et al (2000) Induced posterior vitreous detachment by intravitreal sulfur hexafluoride (SF6) injection in patients with nonproliferative diabetic retinopathy. Acta Ophthalmol Scand 78:687–688

Ono R, Kakehashi A, Yamagami H et al (2005) Prospective assessment of proliferative diabetic retinopathy with observations of posterior vitreous detachment. Int Ophthalmol 26:15–19

Rodrigues EB, Meyer CH, Grumann A Jr et al (2007) Tunelled incision to prevent vitreous reflux after intravitreal injection. Am J Ophthalmol 143:1035–1037

Rodrigues EB, Grumann A Jr, Penha FM et al (2011) Effect of needle type and injection technique on pain level and vitreal reflux in intravitreal injection. J Ocul Pharmacol Ther 27:197–203. doi:10.1089/jop.2010.0082

Rodrigues IA, Stangos AN, McHugh DA et al (2013) Intravitreal injection of expansile perfluoropropane (c(3)f(8)) for the treatment of vitreomacular traction. Am J Ophthalmol 155:270–276.e2. doi:10.1016/j.ajo.2012.08.018

Schneider EW, Johnson MW (2011) Emerging nonsurgical methods for the treatment of vitreomacular adhesion: a review. Clin Ophthalmol 5:1151–1165. doi:10.2147/OPTH.S14840

Sebag J (2007) Pharmacologic vitreolysis—premise and promise of the first decade. Retina 29:871–874

Sebag J (2008) Vitreoschisis. Graefes Arch Clin Exp Ophthalmol 246:329–332. doi:10.1007/s00417-007-0743-x

Sebag J, Ansari R, Suh K (2007) Pharmacologic vitreolysis with microplasmin increases vitreous diffusion coefficients. Graefes Arch Clin Exp Ophthalmol 245:576–580

Stalmans P, de Laey C, de Smet M et al (2010) Intravitreal injection of microplasmin for treatment of vitreomacular adhesion: results of a prospective, randomized, sham-controlled phase II trial (the MIVI-IIT trial). Retina 30:1122–1127

Stalmans P, Benz MS, Gandorfer A et al (2012) Enzymatic vitreolysis with ocriplasmin for vitreomacular traction and macular holes. N Engl J Med 367:606–615. doi:10.1056/NEJMoa1110823

Tagawa H, McMeel JW, Furukawa H et al (1986) Role of the vitreous in diabetic retinopathy. 1. Vitreous changes in diabetic retinopathy and in physiologic aging. Ophthalmology 93:596–601

Takahashi M, Trempe CL, Maguire K et al (1981) Vitreoretinal relationship in diabetic retinopathy: a biomicroscopic evaluation. Arch Ophthalmol 99:241–245

Tammewar AM, Bartsch DU, Kozak I et al (2009) Imaging vitreomacular interface abnormalities in the coronal plane by simultaneous combined scanning laser and optical coherence tomography. Br J Ophthalmol 93:366–372

Thresher RJ, Ehrenberg M, Machemer R (1984) Gas-mediated vitreous compression: an experimental alternative to mechanized vitrectomy. Graefes Arch Clin Exp Ophthalmol 221:192–198

Usman Saeed M, Batra R, Qureshi F et al (2011) Reflux of drug during intra-vitreal anti-VEGF therapies. Semin Ophthalmol 26:357–360. doi:10.3109/08820538.2011.588648

Wang Z-LM, Zhang XM, Xu XM et al (2005) PVD following plasmin but not hyaluronidase: implications for combination pharmacologic vitreolysis therapy. Retina 25:38–43

Wang MY, Nguyen D, Hindoyan N et al (2009) Vitreopapillary adhesion in macular hole and macular pucker. Retina 29:644–650

Zhi-Liang W, Wo-Dong S, Min L et al (2009) Pharmacologic vitreolysis with plasmin and hyaluronidase in diabetic rats. Retina 29:269–274

Index

A. Girach, M.D. de Smet (eds.), *Diseases of the Vitreo-Macular Interface*, Essentials in Ophthalmology,
DOI 10.1007/978-3-642-40034-6, © Springer-Verlag Berlin Heidelberg 2014

Printing and Binding: Stürtz GmbH, Würzburg